I0424381

INTERMITTENT FASTING FOR WOMEN

The beginner's guide, how to practice the intermittent fasting for weight loss, fat burning and how to trigger the process of autophagy.

Hanna Greenberg

Hanna Greenberg

TABLE OF CONTENTS

INTRODUCTION

For women who are keen on weight loss, intermittent fasting may appear to be a great choice, however numerous individuals need to know, should women quick? Is intermittent fasting compelling for women? There have been a couple of critical examinations about intermittent fasting which can reveal some insight into this intriguing new dietary pattern.

Intermittent fasting is otherwise called interchange day fasting, even though there are unquestionably a few minor departures from this eating regimen. The American Journal of Clinical Nutrition played out an investigation as of late that enlisted 16 stout people on a 10-week program. On the fasting days, members expended sustenance to 25% of their assessed vitality needs. The remainder of the time, they got dietary directing; however, were not given a specific rule to pursue amid this time.

True to form, the members shed pounds because of this examination, yet what specialists indeed discovered fascinating were some specific changes. The subjects were all still hefty after only ten weeks, yet they had appeared in cholesterol, LDL-cholesterol, triglycerides, and systolic circulatory strain. What made this an intriguing find was that a great many people need to lose more weight than these investigation members before observing similar changes. It was a captivating discover which has urged a significant number of individuals to have a go at fasting.

Intermittent fasting for women has some significant impacts. What makes it particularly significant for women who are attempting to get more fit is that women have a lot greater large extent in their bodies. When endeavoring to shed pounds, the body consumes starch stores with the first 6 hours and after that begins to consume fat. Women who are following a healthy eating regimen and exercise plan might battle with delicate fat, yet fasting is a practical answer for this.

Intermittent Fasting For Women Over 50

Our bodies and our digestion changes when we hit menopause. One of the most significant changes that women more than 50 experience is that they have slower digestion and they begin to put on weight. Fasting might be a suitable method to invert and avoid this weight gain, however. Studies have demonstrated that this fasting design directs hunger and individuals who tail it consistently don't encounter similar yearnings that others do. In case you're more than 50 and endeavoring to acclimate to your slower digestion, intermittent fasting can assist you with avoiding eating a lot once a day.

When you achieve 50, your body likewise begins to build up some endless maladies like elevated cholesterol and hypertension. Intermittent fasting has been appeared to diminish both cholesterol and circulatory strain, even without a great arrangement of weight loss. If you've begun to see your numbers ascending at the specialist's office every year, you might most likely carry them down with fasting, even without losing much weight.

Intermittent fasting may not be an excellent thought for each lady. Anybody with a specific wellbeing condition or who will, in general, be hypoglycemic ought to counsel with a specialist. In any case, this new dietary pattern has particular benefits for women who usually store progressively fat in their bodies and may experience difficulty disposing of these fat stores.

CHAPTER ONE
WHAT IS INTERMITTENT FASTING?

Fasting, or periods of abstinence from food has been practiced throughout the world for hundreds of years. Intermittent fasting with the goal of improving health relatively new. Intermittent fasting has the characteristic of limiting food intake for a certain period of time and does not need to add any changes to the foods that are eaten. Currently, the most common intermittent fasting protocols are a daily 16 hours fast and fasting for a whole day, this for one or two days per week. "IF" could be considered a natural eating pattern that humans are built to implement and it traces all the way back to our Paleolithic hunter-gatherer ancestors. The model that is currently used in a planned IF program could potentially help improve many aspects of health, from aging to body composition and longevity. Although IF goes against the daily routine and norms of our culture, science can confirm that eating less frequently and staying more time fasting can be the optimal alternative to the normal model of breakfast, lunch and dinner. Here are two myths to be debunked about IF.

- 1 - You Must Eat 3 Meals Per Day: It is normally common in Western society to eat three meals a day but this rule has not been developed on the basis of tests that improve health, but it has become the norm. Not only is there a lack of scientific logic in the 3 meal-a-day model, but recently it has been studied that less meals and more fasting could be optimal for human health. Studies have shown that one meal a day that has the same calorie intake is better for weight loss and body composition than 3 meals a day. This finding is a basic concept that is extrapolated into intermittent fasting and those choosing to do IF may find it best to only eat 1-2 meals per day.

- 2 - Breakfast is the fundamental meal of the day: Many false claims about the absolute need for a daily breakfast have been made. The most common considerations are "breakfast speeds up the metabolism" and "if you have breakfast for the rest of the day you will have less need for food". Well, it has been studied, for a period of 16 weeks, that skipping breakfast did not increase your food intake during the rest of the day. It is still possible to make intermittent fasting protocols while having breakfast, but some people think it is easier to have breakfast late in the morning or even skip it completely and this common myth should not hinder it.

INTERMITTENT FASTING METHODS:

There are several ways to do intermittent fasting and each of them can have a specific set of advantages that make them unique. Each type of intermittent fasting has variations in the fasting-to-eating ratio. The benefits and effectiveness of these different protocols can change from individual to individual and it is important to determine which one is best for you. Factors that can influence which to choose include health goals, daily schedule/routine and current health status. The most common types of IF are fasting every other day, limited-time nutrition and modified fasting.

1. **ALTERNATE DAY FASTING:**
This approach involves the alternation of calorie-free days (food / drink) with days of free feeding and eating any kind of food.

This method has shown interesting results with

weight loss, keeping blood cholesterol levels and triglycerides (fats) in check and improving markers for inflammation in the blood.

The main cause that causes this form of intermittent fasting is that it is difficult to maintain during the days of total fasting.

2. **MODIFIED FASTING - 5:2 DIET**

Modified fasting is regulated by a protocol with scheduled fasting days, however fasting days allow food intake. About 20-25% of normal calories can be consumed on fasting days; therefore, if you normally consume more or less 2000 calories on regular days of consumption, you will be granted 400-500 calories on fast days. Part 5: 2 of this diet refers to the proportion that exists between the days without fasting and days of fasting. So with this regime you should eat normally for 5 consecutive days, then fast or limit your calories to around 25% for 2 consecutive days.

This protocol is excellent for losing weight, body composition and can also help regulate blood sugar, lipids and inflammation. Some studies have shown that the 5: 2 protocol is effective for weight loss, lowers improves markers of inflammation in the blood and shows important signs of improvement in insulin resistance. Taking animal studies, this 5: 2 modified fasting diet has generated a good decrease in fat, decreased hunger hormones (leptin) and increased levels of a protein that is responsible for improving fat burning and regulating fat blood sugar (adiponectin).

The modified 5: 2 fasting protocol is simple to follow and has few negative side effects that included hunger, low energy and some irritability during the initial phase of the program. Contrary to all this, however, the studies have also highlighted improvements such as reduced tension, less anger, less fatigue, a more positive mood and improvements in self-confidence.

3. TIME-RESTRICTED FEEDING:

If you know someone who claims to do IF, odds are it is in the form of time-restricted feeding. If you know someone who claims to do intermittent fasting, it's probably a time-limited diet. This is a type of intermittent fasting that is used daily and involves only the consumption of calories during a small part of the day and complete fasting for the remainder. Daily time-limited fasting intervals can range from 12-20 hours, with the most common 16/8 method (fasting for 16 hours, calorie consumption for 8). For this protocol the time of day is not important as long as you fast for a period of time and eat only in the allowed time period. For example, in the limited feeding program 16/8 a person can eat his first meal at 6:00 and the last meal at 2PM (fast from 2PM to 6AM), while another person can eat the first meal at

12AM and the last meal at 8PM (fast from 8PM to 12AM).while another person may eat their first meal at 1PM and last meal at 9PM (fast from 9PM-1PM). This protocol is meant to be performed every day over long periods of time and is very flexible as long as you are staying within the fasting/eating window(s).

Time-Restricted feeding is one of the easiest to follow methods of intermittent fasting. Using this along with your daily work and sleep schedule may help achieve optimal metabolic function. Time-restricted feeding is a great program to follow for weight loss and body composition improvements as well as some other overall health benefits. The few human trials that were conducted noted significant reductions in weight, reductions in fasting blood glucose, and improvements in cholesterol with no changes in perceived tension, depression, anger, fatigue, or confusion. Some other preliminary results from animal studies showed time restricted feeding to protect against obesity, high insulin levels, fatty liver disease, and inflammation.

The simple application and the promising results of a limited diet in time could make it an excellent option for weight loss and the prevention and management of chronic diseases. When implementing this protocol, it is recommended to start with a lower fast-consumption ratio of 12/12 hours and then up to 16/8 hours.

COMMON QUESTION ABOUT INTERMITTENT FASTING:

What food or drink can I consume during intermittent fasting? Unless you are doing the 5: 2 fasting diet (topic discussed above), you should not drink or eat any food that contains calories. Water, black coffee including food / drinks that do not contain calories can be consumed during a period of fasting. In fact, the right water intake is essential during intermittent fasting and some say that drinking black coffee during fasting helps reduce hunger.

Intermittent Fasting you just want the benefit BENEFITS:

Research on intermittent fasting is in its infancy but it still has huge potential for weight loss and the treatment of some chronic disease.

To recap, here are the possible benefits of intermittent fasting:

Shown in Human Studies:

1. Weight loss

2. Improve blood lipid markers like cholesterol

3. Reduce inflammation

4. Reduced stress and improved self confidence

5. Improved mood

Shown in Animal Studies:

1. Decreased Body Fat

2. Decreased levels of the hunger hormone leptin

3. Improve insulin levels

4. Protect against obesity, fatty liver disease, and inflammation

5.
Longevity

Where intermittent fasting is born

The eating routine you follow while Intermittent Fasting will be determined by the outcomes that you are searching for and where you are beginning from too, so investigate yourself and pose the inquiry what do I need from this?

In the event that you are hoping to lose a lot of weight, at that point you are genuine must investigate you're eating routine more closely, but if you simply need to shed a couple of pounds for the shoreline, at that point you may find that half a month of intermittent fasting can do that for you.

Even though there are a few distinct ways, you can do intermittent fasting we are just going to take a gander at the 24-hour fasting framework which is the thing that I used to shed 27 pounds over a multi-month time frame. The fundamental technique is too quick two times per week for 24 hours, and it bodes well to do this a couple of days separated and it is simpler if you pick a multi-day when you are occupied, so you don't end up diverted by sentiments of appetite. At first, you may feel some cravings for food however these will pass, and as you become increasingly acclimated with intermittent fasting, you may discover as I have that sentiment of appetite never again present you with an issue. You may find that you have great focus and fixation while fasting which is the opposite you would expect; however numerous individuals experience this.

While fasting you can and should drink a lot of water to maintain a strategic distance from parchedness, tea and espresso are alright as long as you take a sprinkle of milk. If you are stressed that you are most certainly not getting enough nutrients into your body, then you should seriously think about a juice produced using celery, broccoli, ginger, and lime which will taste great and get some precious supplement fluid into your body. Even though if you can oversee it, at that point it is ideal for adhering to the water, tea, and espresso.

Whatever your eating regimen is whether its reliable or not you should see weight reduction after around 3 weeks of intermittent fasting and don't be debilitated in the event that you don't see much advancement at first, it is anything but a race and its better to get thinner in a direct manner over the long haul instead of accident shedding a couple of pounds which you will return straight on. After the first month, you might need to investigate your eating routine on nonfasting days and cut out high sugar nourishments and any garbage that you may regularly eat. I have discovered that intermittent fasting over the long term tends to make me need to eat progressively sound sustenances as a natural course.

When you are intermittent fasting for lifting weights, at that point you might need to consider taking a gander at your full-scale nutrients and working out how much protein and starch you have to eat, this is substantially more confusing and you can discover data about this on a few sites which you should invest energy looking into for the best outcomes.

There are numerous advantages to intermittent fasting which you will see as you advance, a portion of these advantages incorporate more vitality, less swelling, a more clear personality and a general sentiment of wellbeing. It's significant not to surrender to any compulsion to overeat after a fasting period as this will nullify the impact picked up from the intermittent fasting time frame.

So in determination just by following a two times per week 24 hour intermittent fasting plan for half a month you will get thinner however if you can improve your eating routine when that you don't want quick then you will lose more weight and if you can adhere to this framework, at that point you will keep the weight off without falling back on any accident diets or diets that are only difficult to stick to.

Understanding Into What is Intermittent Fasting and Its Benefits

Intermittent fasting has progressed toward becoming a remarkable wonder nowadays. Late examinations demonstrated that individuals who attempted it have shed pounds, expanded wellbeing, and accepted to have a long life expectancy. Essentially, intermittent fasting is an example of eating that alternates between periods of fasting, usually devouring just water, and non-fasting, for the most part eating anything an individual need regardless of how stuffing. An individual can eat anything he needs amid a 24-hour time frame and quick for the following 24 hours. This way to deal with weight control is by all accounts upheld by science, just as religious and social practices the world over. Followers of intermittent fasting claim that this training is an approach to turned out to be increasingly cautious about nourishment.

There is a wide range of well known intermittent fasts and hundreds progressively potential varieties. There are two sorts of intermittent fasts that are most fundamental and every now and again utilized. First is day by day fasting in which the individual gets the opportunity to eat once every 20-28 hours inside 4 hours. The second is fasting for 1-3x every week, additionally called exchange day fasting, in which an individual eats anything he needs on one day and quick the entire of the following day.

Intermittent fasting has numerous gainful impacts as tried on creatures like rodents and primates. One study found that there has been a "diminished serum glucose and insulin levels and expanded opposition of neurons in the cerebrum to excitotoxic stress." In 2008, a study on intermittent fasting demonstrated that life expectancy increments of 40.4% and 56.6% in C. elegans for substitute day (24 hours) and two-of-every multi-day (48 hours) fasting, separately, when contrasted with a not obligatory eating routine. What's more, a 2009 study demonstrated that intermittent fasting on rodents improved extended haul survival after ceaseless heart disappointment using professional angiogenic, hostile to apoptotic and against rebuilding impacts.

Scientists alert that just a couple of studies have been done on people who are rehearsing intermittent fasts. The impacts of activity and feast recurrence on body creation are a fascinating yet largely unexplored area of research. There are some positive outcomes. Merely a month ago, the Proceedings of the National Academy of Sciences distributed a study showing that lessening calories 30% multi-day expanded the memory capacity of the older. In 2007, the diary Free Radical Biology and Medicine spread a survey that demonstrated asthma patients who fasted had fewer side effects, better aviation route work and a decline in the markers of aggravation in the blood than the individuals who didn't make quick.

What is Intermittent Fasting?

Intermittent fasting includes rotating periods of dining experience and starvation in which you may eat as much as you prefer amid the devouring yet drink just water amid the quick. The point is to accomplish the advantages of calorie decrease and for a few, use it as a vehicle to shed pounds.

Intermittent fasting should be possible over various days, in exchanging 24 hour periods or day by day. The primary alternative requires you swear off a few or all suppers on at least one days of the week. Every day fasting utilizes 24 hour periods of eating and fasting that start an end in the meantime every day, for instance, quick from Monday 6 pm until Tuesday 6 pm, eat as much as you can imagine from Tuesday 6 pm to Wednesday 6 pm and rehash the procedure. Amid day by day intermittent fasting there is a brief period for eating, more often than not 4-6 hours inside the 24 hour day amid which you can eat as much as you can imagine.

A portion of the things that put individuals off is the

dread that they will be incredibly hungry and not stay on track or don't have the foggiest idea how to fit it into their timetable. This is quite straightforward if you plan ahead of time you get to eat your night dinner at basically a similar time ordinary however at an hour either side depending on if on an intermittent fasting stage or an eating stage. Again with a little planning you can likewise oblige mingling and eating out.

The principal factor keeping numerous individuals from attempting is the dread of being eager. Even though this takes a little resolution and a slight degree of inconvenience, in any case, it is quite simple!

Is Fasting the Right Way For You to Lose Weight?

With every one of the considerable number of eating regimens, practice projects and weight reduction pills available it's challenging to envision that despite everything we have issues with weight reduction nowadays. Nonetheless, as a country, we are fatter than whenever ever. It's getting so terrible that stoutness is turning into an epidemic that is present notwithstanding beginning to impact the economy. Notwithstanding whether you have to lose 10 or 100 pounds, the reality remains that you should quit doing what you are doing and begin accomplishing something other than what's expected.

Fasting for weight reduction is in no way, shape or form another approach to lose the additional pounds, yet it tends to be viable in the light of the fact that it encourages us to end negative behavior patterns in an extremely straightforward manner. One of the main reasons why consumes fewer calories come up short is because we would prefer not to abandon the nourishment that we've developed to cherish. Frequently we need to get out from under a lifetime propensity that can be amazingly difficult to do.

When you diet, the first week, for the most part, goes well since you are still in a "transitory mode." The longer you abandon your old nourishments, the harder it gets, and as a rule, following two weeks we as a whole give because the partition was excessive. This is the reason abstains from food bomb as a long term solution.

When you've encountered this eating routine rollercoaster, at that point fasting may be the appropriate response. It works basically because you don't need to "surrender" on your unfortunate propensities. With intermittent fasting you virtually quick for short periods. Amid your swift, you are on a rigorous eating regimen for 2 to 5 days, and afterward, in your off period, you are allowed to eat what you need.

The fasting periods make a calorie shortage which is the reason it empowers you to get in shape. It is pivotal that you pursue an all-around structured fasting plan; however, since you need to quick for the correct periods and have the right eating routine amid y quick for this to work.

This truly isn't difficult to stick to, and it furnishes

you with the adaptability you should be active with getting in shape. Whenever done correctly it is a unique approach to dispose of the additional pounds, and for most of the customary fasters, it, in the end, prompts substantial life changes - without utilizing resolve to compel the progressions upon yourself. Resolve will take you "that" far. Diets power troublesome transformation upon you. Fasting makes it simple, and it truly works.

What is the intermittent fasting diet

Toward the beginning of consistently, exercise centers are pressed for the initial two months as individuals frantically endeavor to catch up on those new year diet resolutions. Realize that the key is nutrition and finding a methodology that works for your long haul. This is the place an intermittent fasting diet is a particularly exciting option when contrasted with other dietary methods.

So does an intermittent fasting diet work when contrasted with different eating regimens? The appropriate response here is a resonating yes. For instance, utilizing a 16 hour quick will keep your body consuming fat for a large portion of consistently! Also, getting the majority of your calories amid a generally little eating window prevents your body from going into starvation mode and urgently clinging to the muscle to fat ratio. Contrasted with a regular diminished calorie diet, this is a considerable distinction. While any diminished calorie approach will at first lead to fat-misfortune, your body is a powerful machine and will repay by hindering your digestion (the exact inverse of what you need) and clutching muscle to fat ratio.

Is an intermittent fasting diet prohibitive? Any eating routine, by its very nature, includes settling on better nourishment decisions. If somebody attempts to offer you on the flapjack diet, run a mile! Eating trash can never be a decent decision. However, most eating regimens will have you endeavor to eat clean regularly. This is extremely difficult to do and is legitimately connected to winding up eating 12 doughnuts in a single sitting following a long time of hardship! Intermittent fasting additionally includes reliable nourishment decisions. However, it gives you more squirm room. It is hard to eat to much garbage in a little eating window after you have just had your solid nourishment. It lets you eat enough to stop you tumbling off the wagon, however.

Perhaps the real advantage of intermittent fasting is that it very well may be a way of life instead of a momentary methodology. With most weight control plans, regardless of whether you do figure out how to tail it sufficiently long to persuade results will, in general, be trailed by a bounce back that is, an arrival to poor eating and fat addition. By review fasting as a long haul solution, this issue successfully vanishes.

Hanna Greenberg

Intermittent Fasting and the Paleo Diet

You may have known about the caloric limitation to delay our lives, yet did you realize that a more beneficial elective exists as intermittent fasting? Intermittent fasting is an incredible method to keep making increases after you've had some underlying weight reduction with the Paleo diet.

We should go over a portion of the advantages.

Intermittent fasting (IF) builds your fat digestion. For whatever period that you hold your quick to a sensible point of confinement, state 24-36 hours your metabolism accelerates, and it will consume more fats cells as you have prepared it to with the Paleo Diet. Intermittent fasting won't diminish your muscle mass like caloric confinement. Caloric confinement has a progressively detrimental impact with regards to your skeletal muscle, compared to intermittent fasting. Intermittent fasting enables evacuate to squander material. Autophagy is where squander material is expelled from your cells, and this procedure is started by starvation.

Frequently, individuals will in general use IF once per

week because of difficulties with employment, school, and eating socially with others; yet you may do it up to 3 times each week, or littler sessions ordinary. It is best for every individual to choose what works for their body through experimentation. The key is to begin off moderate, so you don't make an early assurance that it is too hard even to consider handling. One strategy is to have breakfast one day, and after that not have again until lunch the following day, or pick another dinner to do this with however you see fit.

Also, there are different advantages to IF. A portion of these advantages incorporate assurance from Alzheimer's illness through the increased production of BDNF (cerebrum determined neurotropic factor), lowering of cholesterol levels and triglycerides increased insulin affectability and increased life span. Other progressively recounted advantages incorporate mental clearness and more grounded protection from stress.

The revelation of life span benefits emerges from an investigation directed on rodents where they were exposed to times of IF for 24 hours, and an assurance was made that their lives were drawn out without affecting the advancement of their bodies and organs.

A fascinating symptom for those Paleo health food nuts which look into weightlifting and exercise is that intermittent fasting can prompt an expansion in development hormone, particularly in men. Development hormone has numerous advantages for grown-ups including increased muscle mass and impacts on the skin which help produce a look of youth. Try not to stress over it influencing your workouts either, studies on competitors who prepared amid times of fasting have demonstrated that it has next to zero impact on their execution. Now and again, it can improve the metabolic parity of competitors to all the more likely separate muscle versus fat rather than muscle.

The Fast Diet

The Fast Diet is the eating plan that enables you to eat the nourishment that you generally expend five days seven days. On two days however not consecutive days amid the week, you lessen your food and caloric admission to about 25% of what you regularly eat. For men, the decrease would convey the day by day calorie admission down to an aggregate of 600, and for ladies, it would be 500 calories every day. The diet is likewise called the 5:2 intermittent fasting diet.

When you don't eat or when you are fasting, the body responds by hoping to put away sources to give the fuel and vitality required for your body to work legitimately. The agency will take advantage of the glucose in the blood for energy. At the point when that glucose is drained the body will hope to put away glucose or glycogen which is created from starches and put away in the liver and muscle tissues. At the point when the accessible glycogen is spent, the body will take advantage of fat stores for essential vitality.

Fasting isn't prescribed for expanded timeframes; with delayed fasting the body will go into starvation mode, hindering its digestion because of diminished calorie admission. On the fast diet, the decrease in calorie consumption or the "fast" period does not last longer than 24 hours.

Even though the research is constrained and a lot of it has not been looked at with studies including people, a portion of the advantages touted with intermittent fasting incorporate decrease of muscle to fat ratio, the deferred beginning of Alzheimer's and dementia and improvement of temperament.

- Studies propose that when you select intermittent fasting, you lose solely fat. While exploring different avenues regarding the diet, creator and doctor Mosley diminished his muscle to fat ratio from 28 percent to 20 percent.

- Studies of mice that are inclined to Alzheimer's and dementia show that fasting can defer the beginning of these medical problems. In examining the ailment inclined mice, they, for the most part, build up the illness about the age of one which is middle age in their life expectancy. Anyway, when they are in a fasting state, the infection is deferred until they are around two which is identical to the age of 90. These outcomes are empowering, yet research studies with people are required. Research with mice indicates intermittent fasting may stimulate the production of the protein in the mind that guides in delivering cerebrum cells in charge of memory. This equivalent protein has likewise been appeared to stifle uneasiness and hoist disposition.

Presently the jury is still out, research connected to

the fast diet has delivered some reassuring outcomes in creature studies. Studies with people are necessary before the demonstrated issues can be noted as apparent advantages of this diet. The fast food limits calorie admission and recommends feast choices that are high in organic products, vegetables, and fiber. Every one of which will complete a body decently and are steady with alternatives suggested for a reliable way of life.

Fasting Diets - Do They Work?

Individuals currently have progressed toward becoming wellbeing cognizant, and a great deal of significance is being given to wellbeing diets and wellness. There are a ton of rec centers that have come up as of late, and people similarly are thronging the exercise centers. To keep up the correct shape and to remain fit, it will most likely require investment and things don't work medium-term. Our food habits and the diet we take assumes a vital role in keeping us fit, and any adjustment in the food we eat can include calories, and we return to our old shape effectively. Extra fat is a common issue, and a considerable number of individuals are large. However, next to no amount of individuals realize that being overweight can prompt questions. In an offer to decrease weight and get into shape, numerous individuals give a shot fasting diet. Do they work? This is an ordinary inquiry, and a few people don't have the appropriate response. Fasting diets can do something amazing just if they are followed in the right way.

You will discover scores of fasting diets, and they don't enable you to quit eating and starve. These diets will allow you to taste and in the meantime won't add calories to your body. Calories are dangerous, and each food we take contains several calories. Eating admirably and practicing the correct way is the fundamental idea of these fasting diets. Green tea is said to be the best thing that consumes calories and keeps you fit. This unique tea is brimming with enemies of oxidants and caffeine. It expands body digestion, and thermo beginning happens in the human body. Green tea is, and it likewise blocks fat absorption into the cells. That way you won't just get thinner yet, besides, don't put on weight with ordinary green tea use. Numerous wellness specialists and diet experts educate green tea as one concerning the fasting diets, and it is a special diet that does some incredible things for you.

Aside from green tea, you can likewise begin intermittent fasting diets. This fasting again won't enable you to starve. You would need to make an arrangement and change your dietary patterns. Amid the time of fasting, you won't eat healthy food yet can take loads of water. Admission of water will keep your body hydrated and avoids queasiness; spewing and you wouldn't wind up frail. A few people quick harshly, and that can be hazardous for them. The blood glucose levels drop, and they may even turn out to be debilitating. That is the motivation behind why you shouldn't starve completely.

Intermittent fasting diets have various types of methodologies. You can quick two times every week and that too for ceaselessly 24hrs. Amid the fasting time frame, you can take water and shouldn't eat anything. Doing this two times every week can enable you to lose 1 to 2pounds. You can pursue another diet where you quick for 16hrs and eat amid the different 8hrs. After the fasting time frame, you can take food that has lesser calories. Eating new foods grown from the ground servings of mixed greens and drinking milk will keep you sound.

These fasting diets would require practicing each week. You can design the calendar and exercise just on interchange days. Hit the exercise center on the day when you take food. If you are fasting, at that point take rest at home. Great arranging will dependably work, and the fasting diets can genuinely enable you to shed the additional fat in your body if you are falling wiped out when you are under a fasting diet, at that point counsel a wellbeing master or a diet expert.

Get in shape - Diets Don't Work, Intermittent Fasting Does!

To shed pounds, you have to consume a more significant number of calories than you are taking inconsistently. Nothing excessively substantial there, I know. The issue that a great many people have when endeavoring to shed pounds is that they make it increasingly troublesome that it should be. If you keep it straightforward and stay with it, you will accomplish the outcomes that you are searching for.

If your eating routine relies upon you checking each calorie, gauging your nourishment, and limiting your admission to the point that you are hopeless, you will stop before any tangible outcomes are accomplished. For an eating regimen to get results, it needs to confine your calories in a manner that is anything but difficult to pursue and enables you to keep up some feeling of regularity in your life. The vast majority of them don't do this, which is the reason I state that diets don't work, at any rate not in the long haul.

As I would see it, intermittent fasting is an ideal approach to get thinner. Before you get too stressed over fasting and feel that you can't do it, let me clarify. Intermittent fasting enables you to in any case eat regularly just as eat a similar way that you ordinarily do. It is far less restrictive than other eating regimen designs and is the best long haul arrangement that I am aware of. If you quick two times every week you will diminish your caloric admission around 20 percent for each week. This will make you lose critical weight just as let despite everything you eat the sustenances that you cherish.

If you typically eat 2,500 calories every day and quick two times seven days, you should cut your calories by around 3,500 every week.

2500 X 7 days = 17,500

17,500 X 20% = 3,500

Three thousand five hundred calories make up a pound of fat which will compare to losing around a pound of fat seven days. Intermittent fasting is a significant haul arrangement and can be utilized for whatever length of time that you like. When you have to lose a little measure of fat, it can assist you with getting lean and have your six pack demonstrating throughout the entire summer. If you have to miss a great deal of fat, you can utilize fasting as long as it takes to achieve your objective. I for one used it to shed around thirty pounds and still quick sometimes to keep up my body under 10% muscle to fat ratio at 41 years of age.

If you imagine that a pound seven days isn't sufficient, reconsider. Any of these cases that individuals can shed 15 pounds in seven days are usually bogus, are for the most part water weight, and are not the long haul. If they worked so well, individuals wouldn't have to attempt ten distinct diets a year and yo-yo their weight here and there without fail. It's the ideal opportunity for you to stop scanning for the following craze diet and put your weight misfortune issues behind you. Out intermittent fasting an attempt and watch the fat soften off step by step.

CHAPTER TWO

PHYSICAL BENEFITS OF INTERMITTENT FASTING

Many intermittent fasting benefits have been found by researchers who need to restrict caloric intake for some reason. Intermittent fasting is depicted as not eating for around fifteen hours. With this technique, many characteristics of the body can be improved. The official inquiry isn't whether fasting can support you, however, how it will help you and how frequently you ought to do it.

This style of fasting has been appeared to lower circulatory strain, and increment HDL levels. It can extraordinarily help with overseeing diabetes, and it will enable you to get more fit too. These impacts sound quite tremendous and can be accomplished with this kind of fasting. Concentrates that have been done on several different species of creatures demonstrate that limiting caloric admission builds their lives by as much as 30 percent.

Concentrates on people demonstrate that it decreases pulse, glucose, and insulin affectability. With these tests, it makes sense that fasting whenever accomplished for an extended period will expand a human's life. Similar outcomes can be achieved by cutting your calories by 30 percent always. However, this has been appeared to cause wretchedness and fractiousness. Fasting is an answer that has been displayed in the spot of essentially cutting calories, and it has the benefits without the gloom or peevishness.

Intermittent fasting works by eating sustenance each other day. When that you do gobble you will finish up eating twice as much food as you regularly would. You are as yet getting a similar measure of calories, yet you get the majority of the benefits too. It will lower stress levels and improve your general wellbeing levels. This kind of fasting is an incredible method to show signs of improving physical condition, to carry on with a more extended life, and to feel better always.

The Wonderful Benefits of Intermittent Fasting

The example of eating called "Intermittent Fasting" as

a rule implies one fast for a timeframe and feeds for a deadline. Many pick a 24-hour cycle of fasting, at that point, eat well the following day and proceed with this procedure as a way of life change.

Research has been done on creatures to discover the advantages of this kind of fasting, and you will be glad to realize it indeed can be useful to your wellbeing!

Intermittent fasting can add 40%-56% more years to your life! That in itself is reason enough to do it. Anyway, different advantages incorporate body weight decrease and fat oxidation.

When you were quick, your body is compelled to search for fuel along these lines expelling matured and harmed cells simultaneously. This kind of purges the assemblage of annoying and undesirable things and helps the weight reduction and advantages of the significant nourishment decisions be expanded and progressively gainful to your body.

Rodents have been appeared to have a long haul and improved survival after heart disappointment after being on an IF eating plan, as well. Specialists are likewise saying that it may help age-related deficiencies in intellectual capacity, as well, with the goal that reveals to me that it may help avoid Alzheimer's Disease and different sorts of Dementia!

Your danger of coronary illness and other heart sicknesses may likewise be diminished when you begin a solid intermittent fasting routine. Your hazard for other interminable diseases and ailments will similarly doubtlessly be decreased.

A more beneficial you can start with intermittent fasting and reliable sustenance decisions! Keep carbs to 50-100 grams every day. Numerous ladies eat between 1200-1500 calories for each day, and when constraining their carbs, they are as yet shedding pounds. Men can deal with up to 2000 calories for each day. Less is ideal, and you have to determine caloric admission dependent on your action, for example, buckling down and working out.

Drink loads of liquids, particularly water and exercise in the nights if conceivable. This will help with those late night cravings.

Once you begin eating and drinking more beneficial, your body won't need to such an extent (assuming any) shoddy nourishment, so settling on reliable sustenance decisions will necessarily get more uncomplicated and more straightforward as you advance in the intermittent fasting schedule.

Substitute Day Fasting or ADF implies long rotating stretches of eating and not eating any sustenance, yet there is likewise intermittent fasting called Modified Fasting where you devour about 20% of your typical calories one day and afterward eat ordinarily (yet sound) the following day. This is frequently progressively achievable for individuals since they feel less denied when they can, at any rate, eat something every day, despite everything it has the vast majority of the advantages of the ADF routine.

Whatever you do, ensure you tell your therapeutic services proficient of your arrangements so the person in question knows and can work with you to achieve your objectives. If you need to get in shape, lose fat and feel much improved, at that point intermittent fasting may be the response for you!

Intermittent Fasting and Bodybuilding: How to Make It Work for You

Is it only a fleeting sensation or is it digging in for the long haul? Intermittent fasting appears to have appeared suddenly in a previous couple of months. Intermittent fasting which is an entirely extravagant (now and again off-putting) state for what is essentially two windows - a window when to eat and a window when not to eat.

Intermittent fasting and lifting weights can work for you if you will probably construct muscle and to get slender and here are three reasons why.

1. Ongoing examinations have demonstrated that it is an established truth all out macros and the aggregate sum of every day calories that represent muscle development and not the measure of meals and the planning of them. Essentially this is stating that as long as you get the required standard of calories in the 24 hours, it doesn't make a difference when you get them. So as long as you understand you required a

measure of calories (an overflow of your TDEE is needed for the mix with a dynamic preparing schedule) in your eating window, you will pick up muscle.

2. One feature of intermittent fasting weight training that individuals whine about is the measure of sustenance and calories that should be expended inside the eaten window. Even though you in all probability should alter if you are right now eating 6-8 little meals daily, over two or three weeks your stomach will conform to eating more substantial meals. I thought that it was tough to eat large meals in the first place; however within a week or so I balanced, and now I have no issues securing large measures of sustenance in one sitting. Take as much time as is required with the adjustment period and don't hope to have the capacity to switch overnight.

3. Keep in mind, such as everything else intermittent fasting isn't an exact science and if you have to expand our eating window from state an eight-hour eating window to a nine-hour window to suit your total calories and dinner necessities, that is fine feel free to do as such. Like any program, it's imperative to discover what works for you. Intermittent fasting, weight training, and building muscle can cooperate,

and its excellence is if you locate that sweet recognize that works for you-you'll get the advantages of intermittent fasting while at the same time keeping up or assembling your constitution to a lifting weights level.

Weight reduction: Intermittent Fasting

The standard eating regimens where you cut your calorie admission amid the whole eating routine, either by reducing the carbs or fats are gradually ending up less well known. Imagine a scenario in which you can eat your preferred sustenance and still lose the muscle to fat ratio.

The Intermittent Fasting diet speaks to an example of eating that switches back and forth between time of not eating (Fasting) and a time of eating (additionally called a sustaining window). The fasting stage is a timeframe where no calories are expended (no one but water can be devoured or relying upon the methodology some thick calorie beverages like espresso). The nourishing window is the point at which you devour entire sustenance. On a more extended term, this sort of eating will make calorie shortfall (eating fewer calories than your body consumes).

As indicated by various examinations there are multiple advantages to Intermittent Fasting. Weight reduction is the greatest one of them. Amid the fast, muscle versus fat is utilized as an energy source rather than put away glycogen. Amid the quick HGH (Human growth hormone which jam bulk and enables consume to fat) is discharged in the circulatory system and furthermore Insulin levels are diminished, which implies that your body will store less fat.

There are couple of ways to deal with Intermittent Fasting:

- Sixteen hours fast, trailed by an 8-hour nourishing window (Lean gains diet).

- Twenty hours fast, trailed by a 4-hour bolstering window.

- 24-hour fasts, a couple of times each week.

Furthermore, there is additionally the Warrior Diet where you can break the fasting time frame by eating little portions of vegetables or products of the soil dosages of protein.

A genuine case of the Intermittent Fasting diet is the Lean gains diet where you adjust between 16 hours fast and an 8 hour bolstering period:

- The fast can start at 8 p.m. Furthermore, last till noon a few days ago.

  Usually, people are dynamic toward the beginning of the day, either by working or doing their morning exercise.

- Noon first and biggest feast - half of the absolute calories

- 4 p.m. second feast - 25% of the absolute calories

- 7-8 p.m. last feast - 25% of the absolute calories

Why You Should Try Intermittent Fasting

Intermittent fasting is a dubious weight reduction system since it includes not eating sustenance for an all-inclusive timeframe. Numerous individuals have the idea that not eating will hinder your digestion and send your body into starvation mode, yet it turns out this isn't valid in any way. The human body was intended to go significant lots of time without eating, so intermittent fasting is a personal practice. Maybe that is the reason it is so viable.

If you might want to get in shape however would prefer not to surrender specific sustenance or would prefer not to share in vivacious exercise, intermittent fasting is presumably your best alternative. Fasting will enable you to shed pounds immediately, regardless of whether you don't eat very sound or activity, although that would extraordinarily upgrade your outcomes. This procedure doesn't expect you to bring down the measure of calories you devour. It just takes a tad of order to start with.

If you don't care for fasting, maybe the benefits will persuade you out it an attempt in any case. Intermittent fasting has numerous benefits that will extraordinarily increase a fantastic nature. A portion of the benefits include:

- Rapid fat misfortune

- Lowered pulse and cholesterol

- Increase in vitality, particularly in the mornings

- Enhanced memory and psychological capacity

These are only a couple of the numerous benefits that fasting can offer you. If you necessarily need to be a more advantageous or potentially more joyful individual, it would be of your best enthusiasm to start an intermittent fasting schedule. Taking everything into account, in what manner may you start?

There are several different ways one can start fasting. One technique, the one I like, is everyday fasting. This includes eating your sustenance for the day inside a timeframe of 6 to 8 hours. This would mean you quick for 16 to 18 hours consistently. The most straightforward approach to do this is to skip breakfast in the mornings. You will profit enormously from this. Considerably more significant benefits will be experienced when you can stretch the time spent fasting. For instance, quick for 20 hours and eat for 4. Make sense of what works best for you.

Another technique that likewise functions admirably is week by week fasting. This would include a time of fasting that lasts between 24 and 36 hours. Along these lines, for instance, you would eat as you regularly accomplish for six days of the week, at that point one day you would not eat any nourishment whatsoever. Drink a lot of water amid when you are not eating. A week after week fasting is additionally successful, however not as powerful as everyday fasting I have found. I urge you to find out more and start to fuse one of these procedures into your life.

Helpful Low Carb Intermittent Fasting

When you are thinking about low carb intermittent fasting, you will need to make a point to peruse the whole section.

Low carb diets may mean constraining carbs to 100 or even 50 grams for every day. This implies decreasing sugars, starches, and all high carb foods. This is better for your body because your pancreas doesn't need to fill in as difficult to expel sugars from your framework.

Intermittent fasting implies fasting for a decided measure of time (numerous individuals quick 24 hours at that point eat healthy the following 24 hours, etc.). This means your body needs to search around for sustenance (fuel), and in the process disposes of awful matured or harmed cells and other waste that has developed in your body.

Consolidate the two of these for "Low Carb Intermittent Fasting," and you'll have a triumphant blend to getting in shape and feeling extraordinary!

When you are fasting, you can, in any case, have low carb and low-calorie beverages, for example, water, and dark espresso, however, you ought not to eat foods for 24 hours. You can eat healthy the next day. However, you should, in any case, keep watch on your carbohydrate admission. Peruse marks and research foods to realize you are settling on the best choices for your body and your wellbeing.

"Live," or fresh foods are always incredible choices. Keep in mind garbage in methods garbage out, and healthy decisions mean a more advantageous lifestyle. This is a lifestyle change and ought to be a steady method for eating for you (at any rate the low carbs). You need to try to settle on astute sustenance and drink choices!

Join low carb intermittent fasting alongside exercise, and you'll be fit as a fiddle before you know it and will feel incredible.

Intermittent fasting diminishes fat oxidation and may lessen body weight. Practicing will speed the procedure along and will enable you to dispose of overweight skin and get conditioned.

Intermittent fasting that has been led on creatures demonstrate a life expectancy increment of 40% or more. That is stunning! This shows how much eating healthy and purifying your body can profit not just your framework and help you get thinner, yet it can likewise expand your days on this planet.

Low carb nourishment choices are vegetables. You can necessarily eat the same number of the plant as you need. Meats and fish are great supper choices. For lunch, you could make a serving of mixed greens with a bubbled egg, onion and a dash of cheddar. Watch the carbs in the dressing, however.

For whatever period that you are resolved to settle on healthy lifestyle choices, your craving for sugars and carbs will no doubt be no more. That craving will be diminished! You'll never again need greasy, sweet foods, when you begin settling on the choice to eat healthy, low carb foods.

Drink bunches of water, as well. Different refreshments that are great are dark espresso and green tea, however, don't try too hard on the caffeine. What's more, recollect before beginning any eating regimen plan or exercise schedule, dependably check with your therapeutic services proficient! You need to ensure you remain healthy while getting more advantageous!

CHAPTER THREE

PSYCHOLOGICAL BENEFITS INTERMITTENT FASTING

1. Weight misfortune

Intermittent fasting may drive weight misfortune by bringing down insulin levels.

The body separates starches into glucose, which cells use for vitality or convert into fat and store for later use. Insulin is a hormone that empowers cells to take in glucose.

Insulin levels drop when an individual isn't devouring sustenance. Amid a time of fasting, it is conceivable that diminishing insulin levels makes cells discharge their glucose stores as vitality.

Rehashing this procedure consistently, similarly as with intermittent fasting, may prompt weight misfortune.

Intermittent fasting can likewise prompt the utilization of fewer calories by and large, which may also add to weight misfortune.

2. The lower danger of sort two diabetes

Intermittent fasting may likewise have benefits for diabetes counteractive action, as it can help weight misfortune and possibly impact different components connected to an expanded danger of diabetes.

Being overweight or corpulent is one of the primary hazard factors for treating type 2 diabetes.

What do the studies state?

A 2014 survey paper in the diary Translational Research analyzed proof that intermittent fasting can bring down blood glucose and insulin levels in individuals in danger of diabetes. The creators state that intermittent fasting or exchange day fasting are promising for weight misfortune and decreasing diabetes chance. More studies are vital.

Among grown-ups who were overweight and fat, the scientists watched decreases in markers of diabetes, for example, insulin affectability.

Thus, they recommend that intermittent fasting could bring down the danger of sort two diabetes in this gathering of individuals.

Nonetheless, a 2018 rodent think about distributed in the diary Endocrine Abstracts proposes that intermittent fasting could expand the danger of diabetes. The examination followed the consequences of intermittent fasting in rodents over a 3-month time frame.

While there was a decrease in weight and sustenance admission, there was an expansion in stomach fat tissue, a lessening in muscle, and indications of the body not utilizing insulin legitimately. These are hazard factors for sort two diabetes.

Researchers need to recreate the consequences of this investigation, and further research is currently essential to see if these discoveries in rodents apply to humans.

3. Improved heart health

Scientists have additionally discovered that intermittent fasting could improve parts of cardiovascular health.

What do the studies state?

An audit from 2016 reports that intermittent fasting could prompt a decrease in circulatory strain, heart rate, cholesterol, and triglycerides in the two humans and creatures. Triglycerides are a sort of fat present in the blood that has connections to a heart ailment.

4. Improved brain health

Studies in mice have appeared intermittent fasting

could improve brain health.

What do the studies state?

One investigation found that mice that were on a concise intermittent fasting diet would be wise to learning and memory than mice with free access to nourishment.

Further research in creatures recommends that intermittent fasting can stifle irritation in the brain, which has connections to neurological conditions.

Other creature studies have discovered that intermittent fasting can decrease the danger of neurological issue, including Alzheimer's ailment, Parkinson's infection, and stroke.

More research is essential to explore whether these discoveries apply to humans.

5. Diminished danger of disease

Creature studies likewise recommend that intermittent fasting may help lessen the danger of malignant growth.

What do the studies state?

A progression of late studies in creatures demonstrates that prohibitive weight control plans, for example, intermittent fasting could postpone the beginning of tumors. Be that as it may, no present studies have set up connections between intermittent fasting and disease in humans.

Obesity is a hazard factor for a wide range of tumors, so the weight misfortune part of intermittent fasting could be in charge of the diminished malignancy chance that a few studies indicate.

Intermittent fasting can likewise diminish a few organic elements with connections to malignancy, for example, insulin levels and aggravation.

There are signs that intermittent fasting could

diminish the danger of disease. Further research in humans is essential to help this case.

Step by step instructions to Fast to Lose Weight Properly.

There are fasting and fasting, and just to quit eating isn't how to quick to shed pounds properly. Everyone needs a specific measure of nutrition in their eating regimen from every day to keep up healthy digestion and insusceptible framework, and keeping your body from both of these essential components of its natural chemistry is to change your life for the sake of weight misfortune.

A few superstars guarantee to have been on detox eats fewer carbs where all they took in was water and fiber to clear their arrangement of contaminations. The main thing that has been experimentally demonstrated here is that they shed pounds. Here, we are examining fasting as a method for getting more fit, and that's it. So how might we quick to get more fit properly?

It is exceptionally undesirable to abandon nourishment totally, for reasons addressed previously. Your body has a specific requirement for nutrition, particularly certain nutrients and plant chemicals (phytochemicals) that help your insusceptible framework and digestion. Without these, you can turn out to be incredibly sick.

Likewise, the contention that by ingesting just fluid sustenances and no solids our body will be compelled to consume fat does not hold water. Every useful part of our eating routine are diminished water and fat solvent fluids, and what powers your body to consume fat is an absence of sugars in your eating regimen, not a lack of healthy nourishment. By the by, by including only enough foods grown from the ground squeezes in your fluid eating regimen, and by drinking around three pints of pure water every day, you ought to have the capacity to get more fit and still devour sufficient supplements to keep up the necessary biochemical procedures inside your body.

Planning for, for example, quick will assist your body with getting the best profit by it. Some keep up that a colon purge will help lessen the impacts of any digestive problems experienced, even though this is easy to refute. Nonetheless, it will make no mischief, so if you trust it will help that it could give you a mental lift.

Additionally, it is significant that you don't stuff yourself brimming with starches before fasting since you will basically postpone or even avoid any weight misfortune for occurring. That isn't how to quick to shed pounds properly. It is significant that quick weight misfortune is additionally sound weight misfortune, and stuffing yourself with sustenance preceding fasting is neither stable nor reasonable.

Nor is complete fasting, taking nothing by mouth by any stretch of the imagination, except, maybe, water. This is probably going to harm your framework by pointlessly denying it of nutrition. Remember your purpose behind fasting - to shed pounds. Step by step instructions to quick to get more fit properly isn't to take no nourishment, yet to constrain your body to utilize your fat stores as a wellspring of vitality to encourage your digestion. You ought to have the capacity to accomplish that while keeping up the admission of sufficient nutrition as to stay away from any changeless or enduring harm to your resistant framework or some other substantial procedure.

So in what limit would it fit for you to start fasting in a stable enough manner to accomplish this? In the first place, you ought to think about your day by day schedule. You ought not to make quick except if you can keep away from any diligent work, or circumstances that could be perilous if you felt powerless or blackout. Fasting influences a few people along these lines, and nor should you quick amid monthly cycle.

Choose if you expect to fast for a long stretch, or just for a few days on end, with eating periods in the middle. If the last mentioned, what should you're eating regimen be between fasting periods? Some consolidate an irregular all out quick with juice fasting, so they, at any rate, take in some nutrition, however here again you must be cautious that you are not putting your center body forms in danger. Your liver needs a level of food to stay practical.

When you are not used to fasting, you will think that it is hard to manage without nourishment for over multi-day however, this is all you may require. If you quick from dawn one day until morning the following day, you won't just give your digestive framework a well-earned rest from which it will profit, yet will likewise have the premise of a substantial weight misfortune program that does not bargain your prosperity. That is how to quick to get thinner properly.

By doing this a few times every month, you will decrease the impact of delayed fasting on your body and furthermore help to expel vast numbers of the poisons developed in your framework. When you break the quick, first take two glasses of salted lemon water to flush the frame out, and afterward eat as typical.

CHAPTER FOUR

THE 5 PSYCHOLOGICAL BENEFITS OF FASTING

Imagine you are going in a wilderness without anyone else and this enormous monkey appears unexpectedly and endeavors to assault you. As of now, your body's battle or flight system activates, and you get these very human powers that guarantee your body utilizes its most extreme potential to endure. Without even intentionally contemplating it, your body will generally settle on the best decision to ensure survival by battling, escaping, or solidifying. Your body discharges an entire cluster of synthetic substances with the goal for this to occur.

Likewise, one's body discharges an entire pack of synthetic substances when s/he is fasting since his/her body is eager. To shield ourselves from the negative symptoms related to keeping away from nourishment for a specific measure of time, our body discharges these synthetic compounds. These synthetic compounds are typically removed after a drawn-out time of fasting which for the most part pursues the "hangry" (hungry + furious) feelings related with deferring a feast.

So in what physiological way does our body change amid fasting?

Neurodegenerative disorders:

In mice, lower dimensions of autophagy brought about more moderate neural improvement and an expansion in muscle versus fat. Additionally, smaller aspects of BDNF are related to memory loss, neuronal death, subjective hindrance, and degenerative sicknesses, for example, Alzheimer's malady. Likewise, explore has discovered that an expansion of ketones secures against neurogenerative disorders.

Memory, comprehension, and learning

An expansion of BDNF hinders memory loss, neuronal death, and personal weakness.

Resting

Research has discovered that fasting following eight days altogether improved members' rest contrasted with their rest pre-fasting.

Melancholy and uneasiness

Fasting has been found to decrease altogether indications of tension for 80% of patients that have endless torment. Likewise, for quite a while, lower dimensions of BDNF have been corresponded with higher burdensome side effects, inferring that more elevated amounts of BDNF are related to lower burdensome manifestations.

Moreover, It is notable that practicing is related with lower rates of discouragement that is because, like fasting, our minds discharge the comparable synthetic compounds described with our body being undermined on account of the physical effort our body encounters.

Stroke

In addition to the fact that fasting reduces the danger of stroke, it additionally decreases post-stroke mind harm. The expansion of BDNF diminished kindled cytokines and expanded neuro-defensive proteins.

Fasting, in a figurative sense, can be considered as a one fix all and protection pill for neurodegenerative disorders, inconvenience resting, wretchedness, nervousness, and stroke, while improving memory, cognizance, and learning.

Despite whether you were quick for religious or non-religious reasons, fasting can altogether improve your psychological wellbeing.

How to Lose Weight Quickly - Can This Be Done?

Getting thinner can be a daunting task for somebody who has not ever needed to follow indeed what they are eating and what the nuts and bolts of absorption are. Outfitted with that sort of learning, regular exercise and a powerful urge to accomplish your weight reduction objectives, you can be very fruitful.

Calories decide fat misfortune. Calories are the measure of vitality in the sustenance you eat. A few foods have a more significant number of calories than others. If you eat a more substantial amount of calories than you consume, you won't lose fat, regardless of what nourishments or sustenance mixes you devour.

Heftiness originates from the way that as a general rule the stout individual devours more calories than he/she uses. Stoutness alludes explicitly to having an unusual high extent of muscle versus fat. It is the primary source of numerous issues like coronary illness, heart disappointment, hypertension, diabetes, joint pain, gout, liver and nerve bladder topic.

Muscle is our most metabolically dynamic tissue. If we are losing muscle, our digestion is lower, which means our body does not require as much nourishment vitality as it did a year ago. Muscle devours a more critical number of calories than fat, advancing progressively proficient digestion, which makes it simpler to counteract weight gain.

Diets that advance transient weight misfortunes can do mental damage. Barely any things are more demoralizing than viewing a 10-or 20-pound weight reduction vanish into 2-or 3-pound trouble. Diets that are too prohibitive reverse discharge furiously. Crash diets can enable you to get more fit rapidly. However, the vast majority recover the weight. A portion of these diets is additionally undesirable and dangerous. Crash dieting isn't equivalent to adaptable discontinuous fasting, where dieters quick for two days every week and calories are cycled. For the most part, the weight loss in a crash diet returns when healthy eating resumes.

Exercise is a critical segment of any health improvement plan. However, it tends to confound make sense of the amount you need and where to begin. Practicing gets your juices streaming and helps accelerate your digestion. Interestingly, studies suggest that exercise may build your appetite at first since you are consuming more calories.

Eat the sustenance that will give you an abnormal state of value sustenance. Loads of veggies, organic products, lean protein, entire grains and HEALTHY fats (olive oil, avocados, nuts, and so on). Eat less and exercise more, and keep at it. In time, your body will rearrange its set point to mirror the new reality you have forced by constant battle. Eating is an impulse which can be controlled; permitting you to see extraordinary advantages in your wellbeing.

Getting thinner can likewise bring down dimensions of triglycerides and even increment high-thickness lipoprotein (HDL) cholesterol, alluded to as "great" cholesterol. What's more, weight reduction can help lessen the danger of osteoarthritis and gallstones. Getting more fit can cost individuals some bone. It resembles the body chooses the skeletons don't need to be as solid when they have less burden to convey. Getting more fit all the more quickly implies losing water weight or muscle tissue, as opposed to fat.

The familiar aphorism of "learning is control" most unquestionably applies to remove the pounds. Monitor your overall calories as well as the sorts of calories, regardless of whether its protein, carbs or fats. Furthermore, most importantly top off the nourishment with regular exercise at the rec center or around your home.

Importance of calories

In any weight reduction, diet calorie tallying can be incredibly chafing. A few health food nuts swear by it and take it somewhat excessively far while others never at any point think about it.

In any case, is it a good thing?

It is a troublesome inquiry because realizing the calorie levels in food can help in adhering to a suggested dimension. The issue can be the point at which you get excessively worried about the number of calories in all that you eat, and it removes the enjoyment of eating decent food.

If you have not been checking calorie numbers on food, at that point, it is an excellent plan to get a thought regarding what the food you eat contains. Doing this will give you a reasonable idea of the nutritional value of your ordinary dinners.

When you have a good thought regarding the run of the mill calorie levels, then you don't need to worry to such a degree. You ought to have a genuinely good idea when you are overeating and can hold it within proper limits.

If you are at the opposite end of the range and are

excessively worried about calorie tallying, then it might be an ideal opportunity to stop...unless you are accomplishing extraordinary outcomes!

Rather than calorie tallying you may get more profit by dealing with your parts and guaranteeing you have a decent and nutritional eating routine every day.

Segment measure is significant as an ever-increasing number of individuals are heaping the food onto curiously large plates and supposing it is alright because the food is solid. Having large segments gets you into the habit of overeating which is certifiably not a good thing. Rather eat littler parts and set aside the effort to appreciate the food.

Another good habit that works for some, individuals is to set up supper designs every week. By doing this, you can get a gauge of the calorie levels, and you don't need to stress over it amid the day. You are allowed to make the most of your suppers because the preliminary work has just been finished.

What's more, you can likewise feel OK with not staying on track 100% as long as you are generally inside the breaking point. If you may abstain from excessive food intake an errand, at that point, there is a good chance that you won't tail it for long so give yourself the most obvious opportunity with regards to progress.

So the key is balance and attempts not much makeup such a large number of standards that will make any endeavor to get fit as a fiddle an extreme errand.

Calories - Why Calories Matter

Calories are inseparably associated with any dialog of the dietary benefits of different sustenance. Various decisions concerning caloric admission can have expansive impacts on general wellbeing. This is the reason it stays essential for everybody to use sound judgment about day by day caloric admission.

What Are Calories?

The calorie is a term used to portray a particular unit of vitality. As a rule practice, this term was supplanted by the joule. In any case, it remains the most famous approach to portray groups of life that are gotten from the consumption of nourishment. Some various definitions apply to this term. Nonetheless, most basic nourishment applications allude to a calorie as the measure of vitality required to raise the temperature of the water. The gram calorie is equal to 4.2 joules.

In less complicated terms, a calorie is an essential measurement for deciding the limit of sustenance things to be changed over into vitality. While many calories have differing utility, one will, for the most part, need to expend enough calories to fuel everyday exercises. This is important for good wellbeing. Notwithstanding, extreme consumption of calories is related to a bunch of unfriendly wellbeing conditions. This is the reason it is fundamental to monitor calorie consumption.

For what reason Are Calories Important?

Calories are the fuel for your body's day by day exercises. You can utilize put away vitality also. How you fuel your body significantly affects yours all out wellbeing. Over the top consumption of calories can result in obesity. There is such an expansive number of prosperity conditions identified with over-consumption of calories. There are likewise positive wellbeing outcomes that can be brought about by expending to a couple of calories. This is the reason it is fundamental to decide a sheltered range for your particular body. This will enable you to monitor your day by day caloric admission to make a sound way of life.

How Can One Calculate Proper Daily Caloric Consumption for Weight Loss or Weight Gain?

Caloric admission will change fundamentally between various individuals. If you have not been monitoring your caloric admission, you may confront some prompt issues. If you are underweight, you should expand your caloric admission. Notwithstanding, it is likewise insightful to work out. If you are checking calories and working out, it is essential to decide what number of calories you consume every day. You won't most likely decisively decide this. It is anything but difficult to choose a comprehensive range. This will enable you to design your day by day consumption as needs are. In case you are underweight, you should eat a more significant number of calories than you are utilizing. This will ensure that your body has enough fuel to meet the day's exercises. If you are overweight, it is essential to consume more calories while eating less. A few people recommend that expending 1500 calories for each day will result in weight misfortune for a great many people.

To get a harsh gauge of your optimal day by day admission, make a free figuring of the caloric expenditure of every action that you play out each day. There are bunches of assets that will enable you to decide your base metabolic rate — adding your base day by day cost to the distinctive exercise exercises that you utilize will allow you to select an all-out figure. You can alter your everyday consumption dependent on this aggregate. It is ideal to steadily move your caloric admission toward the path that you are seeking after. If you need to get in shape, slowly reduce your everyday esteems until you experience weight misfortune. A fast decrease in calories can cause genuine medical issues. If you plan to put on weight, increment your caloric admission somewhat every day.

The Importance of Measuring the Number of Calories Burned

Caloric admission isn't the first vital measurement to think about when endeavoring to lose or put on weight. When you perform exercises, you are consuming calories. As your body accomplishes more, it requires more vitality. This is the reason you should compute your day by day esteems dependent on the number of calories devoured and consumed. This combination of measurements will give you the best thought of the overall effectiveness of your eating routine. You can cautiously change your caloric consumption when you know what number of calories you usually consume. This will enable you to make a caloric spending plan for good wellbeing.

How Calorie Can Protect You from Cancer

If you don't utilize tobacco, at that point the most significant thing, you can do to forestall cancerous growth is eaten well, keep up healthy body weight, and get physical exercise. Tragically when studied under 3% of the populace eats a health-promoting diet that meets the rules for malignant growth aversion, and over 68% of the people are overweight or hefty. Following the standards of calorie thickness will lessen an individual's lifetime danger of creating or biting the dust from cancerous growth and furthermore avert against weight gain, coronary illness, and diabetes.

The idea of calorie thickness, the measure of calories in a particular weight of sustenance, may sound entangled. It's hugely a rule that removes the stress from watching your weight. Put: If you load up your plate with plant nourishment, which contain bunches of water and fiber and very little fat, you'll feel full on fewer calories. Also, that is significant because calorie-thick dinners advance overweight and heftiness, and overabundance muscle to fat ratio is an essential driver of many tumors.

A healthy eating routine is one that contains loads of products of the soil. Over being stuffed with nutrients, minerals, enemies of oxidants, and amazing phytochemicals, they are additionally deficient in calorie thickness. At the point when people select these low-calorie foods people likewise get the opportunity to eat all they need until they are serenely full, they don't need to check calories, and they won't put on weight. Prepared foods, for example, sugar, refined starches, and greasy foods and free oils are exceptionally high in calorie thickness. Eating nourishments that are high in calories makes weight misfortune practically inconceivable. This is because people will, in general, eat a similar measure of the weight of nourishment consistently. Since calorie thickness is consistent when people select from low-calorie foods BY WEIGHT, at that point, they will take in fewer calories.

What specialists have found is if the calorie thickness of the nourishment is underneath 400 calories for each pound, regardless of the amount they ate, they all shed pounds. Between 600-800 calories for each pound, with some moderate exercise, they all shed pounds. Between 800-1200 calories for each pound, people put on weight, aside from those with high activity levels. More than 1200 calories for each pound, everybody put on the pressure. For weight misfortune and malignant growth anticipation choosing the right foods is KEY.

The ongoing American Institute for Cancer Research and The American Cancer Society gives an account of malignancy prescribe that the average calorie thickness of the eating routine stay away from obesity and weight issues to be 550-600 calories for every pound.

Foods that are low in calorie thickness are new

organic products, vegetables, entire grains, and vegetables. Crisp vegetables average around 100 calories/pound, new natural products average around 250-300 calories/pound, boring vegetables/unblemished entire grains average around 450-500calories/pound, and beans/vegetables average around 550-600 calories/pound.

I don't think anybody has to know any of these numbers to eat healthily and carry on with a long and healthy life. It anyway is a much simpler approach than considering calories it utilizes general rules and standards to help settle on healthier decisions. If you need to get in shapeshift towards foods that are lower in calorie thickness, for example, vegetables, natural products, entire grains, and vegetables and decrease the measure of oil, sugar, and refined starches in your eating routine.

Center most of your eating routine on the foods that are low in calorie thickness plant foods (vegetables, natural products, vegetables, and entire natural grains), and you will rehearse the key to long haul useful weight misfortune and disease counteractive action. Go for nine servings per day of new products of the soil and 2-3 servings of entire grains and vegetables for a healthy disease averting diet! Eat more, weightless, and live more!

Figure out How to Calorie Shift

So you have to make sense of how to shift calories and lose a ton of weight? Moving calories is another method for dieting that has turned out to be prevalent, and numerous individuals need to recognize what it is about and how to do it. There is a simple method to do it because there is a site that you can turn into an individual from and just by choosing from more than 30 distinct foods, it will make a feast plan for you that you can print out. This printed supper plan is as of now doing the calorie shift for you. You should pursue the arrangement for 11 days, and you could lose as much as 10 pounds.

What is most significant about Calorie Shifting?

The most significant thing this diet centers around is

that you ought to eat at least four dinners for each day. If you are following their dinner plan and eating progressively littler suppers every day, you will get more fit. You get more fit because your body consumes more calories eating along these lines. Your body's digestion is actuated after you eat, and by eating more times each day and calorie shifting, your body is reliably consuming calories.

Is it difficult to continue doing Calorie Shifting?

Most diets are difficult to remain on them because most expect you to eat less, take in fewer calories, and so forth. The calorie shifting arrangement expects you to eat four times each day, spreading out your dinners each 2 1/2 hours. You are additionally permitted to eat until you feel fulfilled. This implies you will never feel hungry on this diet. Most diets fizzle since individuals are greedy and end up tricking or stopping. Also, since you never feel hungry while calorie shifting, you can bear to change how you eat long haul with the goal that you lose the weight you need to lose.

Avoiding High-Calorie Foods at Fast Food Restaurants

This is an important test, yet it is conceivable! You can make the most of your fast food yet watch your admission of calories.

The most significant "terrible" calories are fat calories.

There are high fats, and there are less great fats. Some are even malicious fats that must be stayed away from regardless.

How would you know which ones are beneficial for you?

You may realize that warmed fats are nothing more than a bad memory when all is said in done. They make materials that grow terrible linings in your veins.

These linings are called cholesterol.

There are additionally two kinds of cholesterol. One is the first sort, and one is the dangerous kind. Warmed fat does not make high cholesterol. It makes the one you ought to maintain a strategic distance from.

To talk about fast food and calorie, fatty foods can mean something very similar. There are these days, many fast foods that endeavor to furnish you with a hearty supper in this manner dodging terrible calories.

They will serve you a new plate of mixed greens (that is immediately arranged and contains fiber-rich raw vegetables and servings of mixed greens, some salt, possibly pepper and oil.) It can be a seed oil, similar to sunflower oil that is likewise exceptionally solid. Try not to eat mayonnaise. No one can tell what it contains.

The bread utilized in most fast food chains gives you just void calories. If you can abstain from eating it, do it. Eat the cheeseburger and the plate of mixed greens. If you need some bread entirely, get it at a cook's shop or in a store where you can discover different kinds of food, perhaps dark colored ones that contain entire grain flour. You can have a milkshake. Milk contains fat, yet most shakes are made of less fatty milk that gives you just a couple of calories. You should avoid milkshakes that contain fake hues or flavors. When they provide a natural product, it is beautiful. The physical product is never calorie rich, and their calories are substantial and few.

The most noticeably terrible thing to eat in fast food yet, besides, the most served are French fries. They can honestly do you a great deal of damage. They are seared in continuously hot fat or oil that is overheated and delivers; therefore, substances that become perilous as they add to the production of disease.

Henceforth, if you can't maintain a strategic distance from to eat in fast food, know about what to avoid: French fries. Eat tapas. They don't have a significant number of calories and fat yet at the same time contain some grain.

Eat the cheeseburger without the cheddar that is pure fat and generally not of good quality.

There is a particular decision in each fast food chain. Pick carefully, since you know which foods you need to keep away from. At whatever point you can include some new natural product, do it. It brings down the effect of fat and substantial calories.

Calorie Shifting Eating - What You Can Take and What Not To

Getting thinner however fasting is awful for your body. It does not just demonstrate its proficiency just for short time range, yet fasting can convey numerous ailments to you too. Sharpness and peptic ulcers are the two most common sicknesses that can jump out at a hard 'health food nut.' The newer method, calorie shifting eating, is the most logical and straightforward method for getting more fit in an increasingly extensive manner.

So you need to know 'what are the sustenance that can be taken in calorie shifting eating.' In this short exchange, we will attempt to make sense of this.

The most significant in calorie shifting eating is that you need not purchase any exceptional sort of nourishment to get in shape; neither would you require any weight misfortune pill. Your menu will incorporate every one of the sustenance that you were eating already.

Do you realize the sustenance pyramid? It enlightens us regarding the diverse sort of sustenance and their necessity in our body. , and they state that our body requires green vegetables in the final sum. Calorie shifting eating is no particular case. You can take vegetables like spinach, tomatoes, carrots, broccoli, cauliflower, cabbage and lettuce as much as you can.

One natural product for each day is likewise suggested. Be it any occasional natural product; you take any of them consistently. Natural products like blueberry, strawberry, apple, mango, and banana will give you much vitality. They contain a lot of antioxidants that will assist you with fighting against the regular maturing process and different sicknesses. Low-fat dairy items are better for your wellbeing. Take white meat (chicken and turkey) rather than red meat (hamburger, pork and so on.). You can pick the lean meat like veal if you genuinely need to.

Sunflower oil, safflower oil, sesame oil contain more MUFA (Mono Unsaturated Fatty Acid) and PUFA (Poly Unsaturated Fatty Acid). They will assist you with reducing cholesterol level and other greasy components. Entire grain blossom is superior to anything cleaned white flour as they hold every one of the supplements of the mother oat.

Liquor, tobacco must be carefully banished from your calorie shifting dietary pattern. Although tea, espresso, and cheap food can be taken in this eating regimen plan, it is more brilliant to keep up a vital separation from them additionally as they contain much cholesterol.

Weight Loss: It's All About Calories

Even though individuals are more wellbeing aware than any other time in recent memory, terms, for example, 'calorie' and 'digestion' are not too comprehended as they ought to be, and many are very new to the significance of sustenance and calorie the board to accomplish weight misfortune.

Calories are a proportion of sustenance vitality. This vitality is drawn from the carbohydrates present in the body and their nonattendance; calories are separated from fat. Subsequently, consuming abundance calories prompts misfortune in fat which thus prompts weight misfortune. Along these lines, monitoring what the number of calories one expands and what name of one consumes toward the finish of every day is of prime significance when one is to accomplish by and substantial wellness.

A significant part of calorie the executives is resting metabolic rate (RMR), which is fundamentally a check of the measure of calories the body consumes while very still. The all-out calories the body utilizes every day is a mix of three procedures -

I) Those consumed as per one's RMR

ii) Those consumed in performing day by day exercises and exercise

iii) Those consumed from the demonstration of eating suppers

Expanding RMR and Daily Exercise

Since most calories are scorched in supporting the RMR, the higher it is, the more calories one will use. The measure of lean mass (for example muscle) that one has expands one's RMR. Weight training ends up significant in consuming calories as it constructs slender bulk and lifts RMR levels. Excessive cardio training, however, can cause lost slim volume and lessening the RMR. A balanced exercise routine including weights is along these lines successful in bringing down calories.

Eating customary suppers

Eating six little suppers daily as opposed to devouring three bigger dinners additionally helps in expanding the measure of calories consumed. Each time you eat supper, the body consumes calories in processing and retaining the feast. Along these lines, eating six times each day rather than multiple times expands the calorie consumption because of increment in feast recurrence. Moreover, eating six littler feels makes you feel more full and henceforth over-eating is maintained a strategic distance from.

Different methods

Aside from regular exercise and keen dietary patterns, calories can likewise be brought down by cooking without oils and utilizing methods, for example, steaming, heating or bubbling as opposed to searing.

A significant propensity that a great many people neglect to instill in their day by day lives is that of perusing names of the sustenance they purchase. By adapting to what number of calories are in every single average nourishment, one can more readily see how to deal with one's caloric admission adequately.

While agonizing over precise sums isn't essential, one ought to get an inexact thought of what number of calories one will consume ordinary contrasted with what number of one should consume to get more fit. Studies have appeared to lose 1-lb consistently; around 500 calories should decrease the day by day caloric admission.

The significance of calorie the executives in accomplishing weight misfortune can't be focused on enough and following the means delineated above should put one well while in transit to a less fatty and more advantageous body.

CHAPTER FIVE

COUNTING AND EXAMPLES OF BASAL METABOLISM

How to get more fit?

A standout amongst the ideal approaches to get in shape is to check calories. So what is a calorie precisely? A calorie is characterized as:

' A unit of warmth comparable to the proportion of warmth required to raise the temperature at one kilogram of water by one degree of one condition weight.'

This term is utilized by nutritionists to describe the vitality delivering potential in sustenance. So how would I check calories? Additionally what several calories would it be a good idea for me to expand when I need to get more fit? To address these inquiries, you first need to comprehend Basal metabolic rates (BMR). BMR is characterized as:

'An estimation of vitality required to keep the body working very still. Estimated in calories, metabolic rates increase with effort, stress, dread, and ailment's

So we should separate this significantly further. Your BMR is fundamentally the measure of calories you have to exist if you did nothing throughout the day. When you have made sense of your BMR, you would then be able to begin to check calories aiming to score lower than your BMR, if you accomplish this, at that point, you WILL get in shape! So let's state you had a BMR of 3500. If you check every one of your calories today and you all out them up to 3000, at that point you will get more fit. If you score over your BMR with 4000 for instance, at that point, you will GAIN weight. As referenced before BMR is controlled by various components which are continually changing; thus your BMR estimations should be acclimated to mirror these elements, for example, movement levels or stress.

It's additionally critical to consider that when you get more fit, your BMR will drop due the way that you have shed pounds and are currently lighter and littler in this way requiring fewer calories to exist. BMR is on a steady yo-yo; thus must be observed precisely for the best outcomes. Government bodies have issued guideline amounts concerning the measure of calories that we ought to expend stay sound. I propose that everybody should make sense of their BMR because those guidelines usually are missing the goal.

The last significant point is this: Try to eat well while tallying calories. In principle, you can get in shape eating low-quality nourishment as long as you score under your present BMR. If you will do that to your bodies systems? People will in general use pre-pressed suppers when on a calorie centered eating regimen since producers unmistakably demonstrate the calorie content. Try not to fall into the device! Cook crisp and live sound!

Controlling Your Metabolism

Weight loss programs keep on being at the bleeding edge of ordinary wellbeing news. Current fashion consumes fewer calories supplant each other nearly as fast as they are made. Specialists and wellbeing consultants are continually recommending strategies for improved sustenance and caloric control. While most eating regimens and wholesome plans hold some an incentive to the average individual, the exact recipe for weight control can be found in the body's standard procedure of metabolism. Eats less themselves are organized for controlling metabolism. The fact of eating fewer carbs is that you are probably going to discover the same amount of achievement by expanding your metabolism. This should be possible by executing some basic and standard way of life decisions.

Your basal metabolic rate is the number of calories your body consumes on a typical day. This rate is affected by such factors as your age, sexual orientation, level of fat, and measure of day by day exercise. While a portion of these factors can't be controlled, it is relatively simple to control others. By focusing on your dietary admission and measure of exercise, anybody can build their metabolism. As the metabolic rate is expanded, a higher number of calories are scorched every day. Join this with a decline in calorie consumption, and you have an effective weight loss methodology. The best part is you can accomplish this without burning through $25 on the following craze diet book!

The least demanding piece of the metabolism recipe to control is your dietary admission. The significant thing to recollect while getting ready nourishment is that calories check. Each calorie you expend past your basal metabolic rate will be put away as fat. Consequently, it is imperative to restrain your calories to just the basics. Notwithstanding viewing your calories, there are additionally sure sustenance that expansion metabolism. Flavors and peppers help you consume calories by requiring your body to diminish its center temperature. Ice water achieves something very similar, requiring an expansion in temperature. Most berries stimulate detoxification activity which likewise consumes extra calories. Executing these nourishments into your eating routine can enable your sustenance to work for you.

Exercise is the other controllable variable of the metabolism recipe. It likewise is by all accounts the most trying for individuals to take an interest in usually. If you likely lose just a few pounds, it might be simpler to keep up a sensible eating routine, and include a couple of long periods of exercise to your week after week regimen. Regardless of how much weight you expect to lose, training gives the quickest effect on your metabolism. Exercise shouldn't be strenuous to be fruitful. For instance, strolling four days seven days for only one hour can consume over a thousand calories. This is what could be compared to two moderate dinners! You can envision how rapidly these calories include over several months.

Metabolism is certifiably not a convoluted science. By inquiring about your basal metabolic rate, you can decide what number of calories you are probably going to consume in multi-day. After you have this data, compute what number of calories you devour all things considered. These two numbers can let you know whether you are working ahead or behind your metabolic rate. If you discover you are behind, steps can be taken to diminish your caloric admission or increment your metabolic rate through exercise. Vegetables, spicy sustenance, and ice water are generally instances of low-calorie choices that advance an expansion in metabolism. Complimenting a reasonable eating routine with a light exercise regimen is a perfect method to control your metabolism, so it works for you. Regardless of how you approach it, regulating your metabolism is a positive flame approach to deal with a reliable way of life.

Utilizing Your BMR (Basal Metabolic Rate) To Lose Weight

The basal digestion rate is the rate at which oxygen is used for different body capacities, when the body is at complete rest, not rest but rather merely loose. Everyone should know their basal metabolic rate all the more so if you are endeavoring to get more fit.

A tall, slim individual has a more noteworthy skin surface contrasted with body weight than a short, forceful individual. Along these lines, a higher BMR is expected to keep up such capacity as warmth lost from the surface, and energy required for healthy development.

Muscle tissue has the most astounding BMR than some other connective tissue in the body. So it makes sense that request would have a 5 to 10% lower BMR than a man due to the more bulk in a man.

Amid the rest, the BMR is decreased by 15 to 20% underneath that of strolling level. Each new decade of life cost around a 5% decrease in basal metabolic rate up to age 25. After age 75, the basal metabolic rate drops roughly 7% every decade. It is essential that nourishment admission is dynamically diminished as every decade passes, shockingly it's usually a different way. We typically eat more sustenance as we get more established and exercise less; this is the thing that prompts overweight and obesity later on throughout everyday life.

To get thinner and keep it off, we should build our metabolic while devouring the best possible kind of foods that will fuel our metabolic.

Eating a well-adjusted eating regimen comprising of crude products of the soil will consequently expand your digestion. Foods high in fiber additionally have the additional favorable position of expelling dangerous poisons and development squander from the body. Texture likewise gives you the sentiment of being full and will keep you from overheating. Thread is additionally significant for moving sustenance that has not been processed the majority of the colon. Plant-based foods are high in nutrients and minerals complex carbohydrates, and protein yet is low in calories.

Plant-based foods will build your BMR by opening up vital energy regularly used through processing a high fat and high substance protein diet. If there is more energy available to your body, at that point, this can be used for consuming fat in the tissue of the body.

Checking Calories - Best Way to Lose Weight

One of the best and most robust approaches to shed pounds is by including the calories in the foods you expend. A calorie is a unit of energy estimating how much power the foods we consume give to our bodies. A specific measure of calories is fundamental for the body to work legitimately. As you eat sustenance, your body transforms that nourishment into fuel and consumes it, delivering calories, or energy.

As we all in all know, there are three distinct kinds of foods, all of which have diverse caloric sums: carbohydrates, proteins, and fats. One gram of sugar contains four calories. One gram of protein contains four calories. However, one gram of fat has nine calories, more than double the sum found in protein or carbohydrates. This might be a piece of the reason fatty foods appear to top us off so rapidly. Sadly, it's additionally the reason fatty foods make us put on weight quicker.

The full name for calories is "kilocalories." When

calorie counts are made, it is expected that everyone realizes that calories = kilocalories. For instance, if something on a menu is recorded as having 500 calories, it truly has 500 kilocalories. A calorie is the measure of energy it takes to expand the temperature of one gram of water by one degree Celsius. It takes 3500 calories to approach one pound of body weight.

These numbers and figuring's might make your head turn. Recall, all you genuinely need to know is in the last sentence of the previous passage. If you need to lose one pound of put away body fat, you should consume off 3500 calories. When you're unwinding, doing absolutely nothing by any means, researchers state that a great many people consume only 50 calories 60 minutes. So it usually pursues, at that point, that to make an exact imprint into your body fat, you should join checking your day by day calorie consumption with exercise.

A few people eat various kinds of foods on an eating regimen, believing that will assist them with losing weight quicker. Low carbohydrate consumes fewer calories are famous, as taking in fewer carbs will make the body absorb more protein by changing over protein to sugars in the liver. This can likewise make increasingly liquid be lost from the body, however, faking dieters into supposing they're losing large measures of weight when, in reality, they are merely losing liquid and not making a detectable, lasting decrease of the majority of their put away body fat. This is the reason consumes fewer calories that limit just particular kinds of foods usually don't work.

Specialists express that the best way to get more fit is to build one's basal metabolic rate, usually through vigorous exercise. At the point when a body is very still, the body's oxygen supply is adequate to wreck to 90% of its energy as fat. Therefore, if you increment your resting metabolic rate, you will consume a more significant number of calories very still than the individual beside you. This will push you, and you should see the numbers on the scale decline also.

What is Your Basal Metabolic Rate?

Your Basal Metabolic rate (BMR) is the number of calories your body consumes multi-day while in a resting state. Your Basal Metabolic Rate is a component of your Gender, Age, Height, and Weight. This number is the number of calories that you would consume if you didn't do anything however sit on the sofa and sit in front of the TV throughout the day. As a rule, If you are a Male, your BMR will be higher than a Female's BMR. Additionally, being more youthful, more substantial, or potentially taller will expand your BMR.

Your Basal Metabolic Rate (BMR) is a significant weight reduction metric for two primary reasons.

Most importantly, if you eat fewer calories than your BMR, at that point, your body will quit working appropriately, and it will begin to crowd fat for some other time. This is what is commonly alluded to as going into "starvation mode." At the point when your body goes into the starvation mode, you can anticipate lower energy, slower fat digestion, and physical fatigue. A few people imagine that they have to eat a couple of calories as conceivable to get in shape. In reality, you should go for your BMR or directly above, or else you will rapidly go into starvation mode.

The Second motivation behind why you need to comprehend what your BMR is that you can utilize your BMR to appraise the number of calories you are consuming the multi-day. You can duplicate your BMR by a dimension of activity multiplier which will accurately evaluate the number of calories you consume in multi-day. For instance, if you have office work and don't work out, you consume about 1.2 occasions your BMR. If you work out around three times each week, you consume about 1.55 events your BMR. When you see what number of calories you consume in multi-day, you can design you're eating regimen to enable you to achieve your wellness objectives.

If you need to get in shape, you have to anticipate eating many calories that are somewhere close to your BMR and the total number of calories you consume in multi-day. If you need to put on weight, you have to eat a more significant amount of calories than you consume in multi-day.

CHAPTER SIX

CONSIDERATION OF MACRO AND MICRO NUTRIENTS

Nutrition is the arrangement to body cell and another segment to help life. It is a segment that is basic for the development and advancement of our body. An appropriate amount of nutrition gives all around created safe framework that helps in shielding us from various kinds of illnesses. The examines have demonstrated that the day by day admission of a perfect amount of supplements give us sound living and help us to battle against poverty and appetite.

If nutrition is so much important, at that point, we should examine increasingly about it.

Nutrition is an immense theme that covers the information of an extensive amount of minerals, nutrients, and other essential elements. Supplements can be ordered into two gatherings full-scale supplement and miniaturized scale supplements.

- Full-scale supplements sugars, protein, and fats

- Smaller scale supplements minerals and nutrients

- Full-scale supplements

These supplements are necessary to keep up the structure of our body. Sugars are said to be the repository of vitality. They free starch and glucose that are imperative for the ordinary working of our organization. Proteins are bodybuilding materials that help in the development and advancement of our bones and muscles. Fats are likewise fundamental, as they store and free vitality when required.

All these three mixes sugars, proteins, and fats are the mixes of carbon, hydrogen, and oxygen in various proportions.

Miniaturized scale supplements

It comprises of minerals and nutrients. Both of these substances are important for giving insurance to our body framework. Inadequacy of any of the metal or nutrient can make ailment or lead debilitated insusceptible framework and sick mental wellbeing.

It has been seen that every single of them are essential to finish our eating routine arrangement.

- Nutrition classes

- Vegetables

- Organic products

- Dairy items

- Oats and heartbeats

- Poultry, fish and meat items

Every one of the previously mentioned nutrition types has its claim nutritional esteem. Keep in mind the best possible amount of calorie admission is a must from every single of this gathering. Subsequently, you have to devour these nutritional categories in an appropriate amount. It is a direct result of this reality that it is recommended to go to the nutritional crusade. It causes guardians to able for the proper amount of supplements to their tyke.

Nutrition-related ailments

The ailment can be caused either by overnutrition or insufficiency of nutrition. Taking nutrition in excessive amount can result in the accumulation of fats in our body. It can even prompt a cardiovascular issue. Give it a chance to be over utilization of iron or nutrients; every one of it has its very own disarranges identified with it.

Any of these parts, whenever expended in less amount, can likewise be the reason inadequacy infections in our body. Beri, scurvy, frailty, and thyroid are some of such diseases.

Investigating the above-expressed proclamations, it is must to have appropriate admission of various nourishment segments to have both physical and mental development. Henceforth, it becomes utmost important to not to disregard this issue it is possible that it is for you or your children. In this manner, show your tyke the smart dieting propensities and give him the correct assurance or obstruction against ailments.

The Nutrients Required For Muscle Building

For us to construct our muscles successfully, we require the correct equalization of nutrients to encourage the muscles. We need calories to fuel our bodies every day, and when we work out, we require a higher number of calories than the average individual. It is assessed we need 50 calories for each kilogram of body weight so for an average measured jock that could be 4000 over calories.

Presently we know what number of calories we have to know where we get these calories from, the calories will originate from protein, sugars, and fats which we class as large scale nutrients and the other key component of our weight control plans are miniaturized scale nutrients. In this part, we will talk about the miniaturized scale nutrients that we require.

Smaller scale NUTRIENTS

Our bodies after exercise require nutrients and minerals for vitality and the fix of harmed muscle strands. When we work out, we will need a higher amount of these nutrients and metal than the average individual.

Nutrients

Cell reinforcement minerals are by a wide margin the essential minerals our bodies require so such nutrients of A, C, E, and K. These nutrients will fix the harmed cells that happen because of activity because of oxidation. Oxidant happens in regular day to day existence. However, we require more nutrients as the oxidation is more prominent amid exercise. Products of the soil are the best form of nutrients A, C, and K whereas nuts and eggs are high in Vitamin E.

Remember nutrients B-complex which can be found in nuts, beans, eggs, and hamburger. These nutrients are useful for the fix tissue and creation of red platelets just as making vitality.

Minerals

Minerals are another critical component for any one manufacturer, and they help the safe framework, our vitality creation and capacity of our hormonal structure. The most important minerals for lifting weights are zinc, iron, and calcium.

Zinc-Involved in a fix just as the building of muscle and in the generation of vitality for our bodies. A very much adjusted eating routine which incorporates fish, entire grains, poultry, and veggies will sufficiently include zinc for your requirements.

Iron-is is known to the formation of the substance that will convey oxygen in our blood. Clearly without sufficient oxygen in our blood will make us tired and influence our performance. Incorporate sustenance, for example, fish, poultry, eggs, and beans to guarantee you get enough Iron.

Calcium-is required to keep up our bones and decrease the danger of stress cracks. The most straightforward approaches to get calcium is from dairy items, for example, milk.

Composts and Nutrients

Plants need a scope of essential nutrients to develop well. The measure of compost you use and how regularly you have to apply it will rely upon your dirt and the kinds of yields you are endeavoring to develop. In nature a wholesome cycle happens whereby plants accept nutrients from the soil as they grow, at that point, in the end, bite the dust and spoil, enabling the nutrients to come back to the dirt. In the greenery enclosure, you can emulate this procedure somewhat by reusing all your natural waist in a fertilizer receptacle and utilizing the manure to return nutrients to the dirt. An extent of the fundamental issue isn't answered, so the earth needs recharging from different sources.

Composts are a helpful technique for giving the nutrients that are required for sound development. Your decision will rely upon the nutrients effectively accessible from your dirt and the kind of event you need to empower. There are three large scale or essential nutrients, nitrogen, phosphorus and potassium, the extents of which are communicated as a proportion of NPK on the names of manure packs. Every full-scale supplement promotes another sort of development. Nitrogen encourages verdant development, so it is valuable for including a green harvest, for example, spinach and cabbages.

Phosphorus is an organic supplement for sound roots. It likewise promotes the maturing of natural product. Accessible as potash, potassium promotes flowering and good sustenance production. Three different nutrients, calcium, magnesium and soleplates, are required in littler amounts and are known as optional nutrients, and seven more are additionally fundamental yet in little sums. These are known as smaller scale nutrients or follow components. If they are to flower dependably a seemingly endless amount of time after year, perennials and bushes, for example, the camellia, ought to be given the nutrients they need. Manure wealthy in potassium encourages good flower production.

Genetic material, for example, all around spoiled patio nursery fertilizer or farmstead excrement is high in nutrients — the fork in when the dirt is burrowed. For heavy soils, this is best done in the fall. When the earth has just been borrowed, the natural material can be delicately forked in or left superficially. The worms will finish the errand of working it into the dirt. In harvest time, and again in spring, top dress established plants with a layer of all around decayed natural material. Good patio nursery manure is dim dark colored, stringy and brittle. It has a sweet, hearty smell, not a decaying one. Fertilizer can be utilized straight away or left secured until required.

CHAPTER SEVEN

HOW TO SET UP THIS DIET IN A CORRECT AND LASTING WAY

How would you approach keeping a diet diary? Most importantly take some time after your last meal consistently, or follow along while you are having your meals. Record what you eat and around how much. You don't need to gauge it, only a rough sum. Do this at some point every day of the week or after every meal. Goodness, remember the snacks as well. You truly need to monitor those.

After the week is up, it's an ideal opportunity to investigate your diet diary. Here's the piece of keeping a diet diary that will enable you to perceive how you are genuinely eating; this is the place the recording device model comes in. You get the opportunity to hear what you seem to like, or for this situation how your diet truly piles up to solid food. If you are overeating extended partitions? Are there things that transpired amid the week that made you eat more? Did you skirt a meal one day and afterward eat a lot at another meal that day as a result of it? You don't have the foggiest thought regarding that a portion of your dietary patterns are indeed issues that are correctable once you see it recorded as a hard copy.

The following thing you can do is take a gander at every day of your diet diary. Keeping a diet diary will assist you with realizing what you are fouling up and think about what you can do to address it or limit the issue. If you understand that you don't have ample opportunity to fix breakfast several days amid the week, possibly fix something the previous night. Make a few eggs and warm them up in the first part of the day or feel free to pour a bowl of grain so it will be prepared the following morning. Keeping a diet diary will assist you with resolving issues that are shielding you from getting in shape. Rehash the examination of every day and attempt to explain any problems that you see with the meals you are eating.

Keeping a diet diary for a couple more weeks until your concern regions are resolved will be extremely useful to you.

Another way of keeping a diet diary will be useful in planning your meals ahead of time. Rather than recording what you ate every day or after every meal, plan seven days what you will eat. Put a checkmark close to the meals you eat to ensure you're sticking to your plan. If you plan, this will likewise assist you with creating your shopping list. Just purchase the food for the meals you have prepared to get ready. If that other food isn't around, you won't almost certainly eat it. No longer of any concern as the adage goes. Keeping a diet diary is an incredibly supportive instrument for your diet. You might be astounded how you sound.

Calorie Cycling: Set Up Calorie Cycling in Your Meal Plans

In case you're hoping to jump on a bulk building program while limiting any fat picks up that join it, calorie cycling is a great thought. The idea driving calorie cycling is that as opposed to eating the equivalent extremely high-calorie consumption on all days as you approach your mass structure diet plan, you will shift back and forth between higher calorie days and lower calorie days.

In doing as such, you'll help keep away from any fat

overflow that may happen with a progressively customary mass structure diet plan, along these lines expanding your general level of results.

How about we investigate the fundamental advances that you have to know to guarantee that you perform calorie cycling effectively.

Set Your Weekly Calorie Target:

The simple initial step to execute calorie cycling into your mass structure diet plan is to set your objective calorie admission for the week. Since you will have those low-calorie days in there, you should ensure that on a week after week premise, despite everything you will be in a calorie surplus as this is the thing that will bolster mass structure.

If you aren't, at that point, you're only going to remain a similar size or may even start to lose body weight.

So decide what number of calories over maintenance

you need to be (typically 2000-3500 is a decent range) and afterward duplicate your maintenance calorie consumption by seven and add that number to it. This is your week by week calorie target.

Decide High And Low-Calorie Levels:

The following stage for setting up calorie cycling in your eating routine is to set up those low and high-calorie days. You ought to put the high-calorie days on the days that you are doing your weight lifting exercises since this is the point at which you will be in prime mass structure.

Separation up the calories any way you see fit, making a point to bring those exercise days a lot higher while the off days are much lower.

Try not to go excessively sensational here anyway as you would prefer not to twist up totally starved on the low-calorie days and afterward cheat and ruin the set-up. When concentrating on mass structure, you should keep the quiet calorie days directly around upkeep level or somewhat lower in your calorie cycling diet plan.

Center Carbs Around the Workout:

Next, while organizing the high-calorie days, you ought to likewise ensure that you're setting a significant bit of the carbs you devour that day directly around the exercise time frame.

This is the point at which the body is destined to use them to fit the bulk building, so when you need to benefit as much as possible from them.

You don't need to put all the carbs right now. However, most by far of them should go inside a few hours after completing that exercise for best outcomes.

Keep Low Days Higher In Fat:

At long last, the last point to remember when setting up your calorie cycling mass structure diet plan is to keep the smaller days marginally higher in solid substance.

Since you will put more carbs on the high-calorie

days, it's okay for these to descend in dietary fat so you can boost that starch admission (protein will remain consistent crosswise over both days), yet then on the lower calorie days, raising the fat slightly will go far towards averting hunger improvement.

Besides, it will guarantee that you get all the sound supplements that you need into your body to help mass structure and by and abundant health.

To ensure you remember these focuses as you approach planning a calorie cycling diet. If you do, at that point, you ought to have no problem seeing the great benefits that this eating regimen brings to the table.

Dieting - The Best Way to A Balanced Diet

Nature is a top supplier with regards to the provisions the body needs to look excellent, reliable and stable. One ought not to comprehend diet as a food restraint, yet as a controlled and balanced food admission; an inclination for a specific gathering of foods over those which produced the irregularity.

We should take a couple of precedents: Sodium is an essential part of the well working of the system. Its absence results in various sort of sicknesses, for it safeguards the body against poisons by killing them through sweat. It is additionally useful in modifying the body temperature, much the same as fat. The last is your body's standard cover which protects it from low temperatures. It might come as an astonishment. However, objective measures of fat have the motivation behind keeping up the skin looking great and conditioned. It is likewise a wellspring of oil for individual pieces of the body. Its primary use is characterized by the way that fat is a real storehouse of vitality, keeping your body moving advances after every one of the supplements are consumed. Even though they are should be avoided by many dieting plans, both fat and sodium are required in your life form, as long as the sums are directed. Whatever is the nature of your day by day food admissions, if you have a lot of any supporting food, the result isn't great.

The essential principle of right dieting moves toward becoming not what you're body synthesizes in the metabolic procedure, however the way and extents by which the foods are brought into your system. Take sugar for instance. Expanding the handled sugar you obtained, will give you a quick wellspring of vitality. In any case, you'll see that supplanting it with regular sugar from organic products, and the energy will last longer for your body signs it in slower sums. Abundance must be avoided with espresso also. Toward the beginning of today should have is incredible for giving cancer prevention agents and not just. These components are the establishment of your immune system, keeping your body stable and lively, and furthermore battle against the maturing procedure. A day by some espresso is broadly suggested, yet ingested in bountiful sums, the majority of its advantages evaporate, for potential sicknesses and uneasiness.

Constraining yourself to fitting admissions of food is an ideal approach to have a balanced diet. In case you're curious about the right proportion set in your body's best enthusiasm, there are food graphs accessible to enable you to decide the right amount of each supplement. It's anything but difficult to improve your wellbeing by following the rules of this basic, yet informative food graphs.

In the endeavors of finding the best items to coordinate in a balanced diet, a few people purchase extremely costly foods which ensure a sound and satisfactory wellspring of supplements. In any case, that doesn't imply that everyone must discharge their wallets for being robust. There are a lot of choices accessible at your neighborhood store that could supply your body with whatever it needs, without the additional expenses. For whatever length of time that you realize how to adjust the fixings, you'll sustain your body well, with single contrast living in the cost.

If there's one thing that your body couldn't develop feel worn out on, it is water. You can devour as bounty as you need, without turning into a danger to your wellbeing. Any additional measures of water will, in the long run, be wiped out through perspiration or flushed out.

Accomplishing a balanced diet does not force any

challenges as long as you have an assortment in legitimate sums. In case you're griping of such a large number of pounds than wanted, you can mostly avoid consumption of the foods that you eat most or decline the favored amount until your weight returns to ordinary. And furthermore, include bunches of water.

5 Easy Things to Consider Before You Go on a Diet

Here are five factors that I would advocate while considering going on what we for the most part call 'a diet.'

Work in a Structured Environment.

1. We tend to work better with the structure to our lives as this unites our activities into a propensity. If we following a diet that has some structure to it we have a more prominent possibility of being fruitful giving the establishments of the food pursue healthfully robust standards.

Set Your Expectation Levels.

2. Set our anticipation levels right in terms of how

quick we need the weight to fall off. If you as of now weigh 170lbs are you are hoping to lose 28lbs in your first seven day stretch of dieting at that point overlook this thought straight away. The slower you get thinner, the more shots you have that this weight will stay off. If you set your desires excessively high, at that point you will be progressively disillusioned when you neglect to accomplish this outcome, he could be de-spurring and damage your odds of achieving your objective weight.

Incorporate Rotated Exercise Plans Into Your Life.

3. Incorporate various exercises into your diet plan as one of the central components that you will pursue. Just as firming up your body and building conditioned muscle exercise as different other gainful characteristics, for example, mitigating pressure, the advantages of regular practice can't be over overemphasized. If you pivot the activities that you don't just will you stop the fatigue of reiteration you will likewise not enable your body to become accustomed to the routine?

Take Photographs of Your Progress.

4. Snap a picture of you previously, amid and after your time of dieting. The advantage of this is more

often than not 'scale weight' isn't recounting to the entire story. When we incorporate a weight training routine into our diet, we will lose fat and building muscle. As muscle gauges more than fat we will lose fat and picking up muscle and the scale may be climbing. By having something visual to follow out advancement we can see the progressions create and have an assessment of our progress from an alternate point of view.

Consider Your Diet a Lifestyle Change

5. If you adjust to incorporate exercise into your life and to eat nourishments that advantage you from a healthful point of view, then you will see the outcomes enduring longer if you see it as a way of life change and another method for living. Mentally you won't see this as a short term quick fix solution, and you will permit a more significant level of persistence before you see the outcomes you want.

The creator does not hold any therapeutic capabilities but instead would encourage you to counsel a certified proficient before you set out on any diet and exercise routine.

Real Weight Loss For Real People - Diets Alone Don't Work.

Give us a chance to confront reality, and if it were anything but difficult to change your diet and dietary patterns, there would not be any overweight individuals on the planet. There are incredible diets out there, and vast numbers of them help shed pounds securely. In any case, can the average person stay on a diet sufficiently long to change profoundly instilled dietary patterns and longings? I state no!

- First-disregard dieting...done. That is how most got overweight in any case.

- Second - possibly eat when you are hungry...done. That is how most got overweight in any case.

- Third-illustrate what you need to look like...Does your mental picture have Twiggy chuckling back at you?

- Fourth-when you get the munchies, eat an apple... Finally check an apple was not oily and salty.

- Fifth-Set your treadmill to a 15° edge and walk 20 minutes...In your extra time with your extra vitality, did anyone get overweight by practicing usually?

Most everyone realizes that to have enduring weight loss that you will need to change a few propensities (a ton of inclinations). The main issue is that starting to eat less restricts eating so much that you tumble off the diet before you ever lose any substantial weight. Second, if you attempt to change only one seemingly insignificant detail at once, you don't perceive any progressions and surrender before your body changes by any means.

Thin individuals eat uniquely in contrast to us progressively adjusted people. I made sense of it as of late when my slim closest companion said: "It doesn't care for I never eat the wrong things, early today I had an English biscuit with spread on it!" I can eat that while choosing what to have for breakfast.

Eating is a habit, similar to smoking or liquor misuse; our bodies hunger for sustenance. There is a broad scope of reasons why individuals overeat and additionally, are overweight, yet the main concern is we as a whole need some additional assistance. A few of us don't have the sentiment of being full anymore; we need a reminder to let us know our stomachs are full. A few of us, for different reasons, don't consume the calories how we should. We need a couple of fewer calories without starving ourselves. After some time a few of us have manhandled our digestive systems to the point they don't acclimatize supplements effectively, we need a wipeout and some inside upkeep. A few of us need to discover a substitution for the "in a hurry" low-quality nourishment gorges. Help for every one of these issues is here.

CHAPTER EIGHT

DIFFICULTY OF INTERMITTENT FASTING

Intermittent Fasting - A Way to Lose Fat

Picking a right weight misfortune plan is always a troublesome undertaking and it progressively troublesome when you are doing this at you possess and not taking the conference from any dietitian or any specialist. You may feel that is alright, starting now and into the foreseeable future I am not going to eat I will take once every day, and that is it. To some, it's sound, and to numerous, it sounds a significant errand not to eat anything throughout the day. Need to tell those individuals who state fasting is excessively troublesome, it would be ideal if you note that fasting with the help of expert individuals has an expansive impact on your hormonal parity, it will be extraordinary assistance in losing and looking after weight. You may state that most natural rule for fasting is having ultimately "No Calories At All."

Am I not catching our meaning here by fasting? Exceptionally basic, I intended to state that no having in the middle of your morning meal, lunch, and cafe. Pull out all the stops for 24 hours. You limit yourself to eating in the middle of your three meals. For 2-3 days in the first week do this way. Next week, minus one meal have just breakfast and supper just and no lunch. Again do this second practice for 2-3 days in the second week. You will surprise to see the outcomes.

In the middle of your meals, drink a great deal of water to battle carvings. Diet soft drinks likewise can give flavor to your mouth without breaking the quick. Tea is a natural way to get a taste without calories. Keep your self-purchase always, center around your activity, don't consider yearning and fasting which you are doing. The craft of concentrating on what you're doing which is significant for accomplishing your objective of diminishing additional fat from your body. This is a reality that, we needn't bother with sustenance always, we are accustomed to having it regularly.

You can discover data and different ways of intermittent fasting for weight misfortune however what I am endeavoring to tell here is intermittent fasting that implies ceasing and beginning eating at sporadic interims since it is significantly more potent than some other sort of fasting.

Your body is intended to sustain off additional fat when nourishment isn't available. Exploit this natural framework. Picture the life of individuals precisely 200 or 300 years back when they didn't have general stores and departmental stores and cheap food. They depend on their three meals consistently, and that is it. Envision the life of seekers when they make the thing to eat when they chase down something and after that hang tight for the following chase. Though if you analyze the life of the present man, when he has several choices available for eating, really we made our life hopeless regarding overeating.

Intermittent fasting is especially typical and unbroken, and even it is pleasant, above all, it works when somebody sticks to it for a particular timeframe for losing his additional weight. You won't make sense of the consequences of like this of getting more fit unless you give an attempt, so there is nothing to lose, one ought not to delay out it a struggle.

Intermittent Fasting: A Way to Lose Weight

Wellbeing is riches. It is portrayed as the ideal prosperity of an individual whether it is physical or mental. Remaining fit and solid advances an inspirational standpoint and keeps up a young and dynamic manner. In addition to the fact that it preserves youth, it likewise drags our life. Presently, a standout amongst the most innovative ways to keep oneself sound and fit is through intermittent fasting. If you need to safeguard your wellbeing, youth and the essentialness of your being; at that point, intermittent fasting ought to be given an attempt.

Intermittent fasting, as depicted today, is one of the least expensive fasting diets to get more fit. It doesn't require some other devices, for example, pills or meds, nor does it involve any costly rec center hardware. All it asks is a precise and stern control to fasting. Intermittent fasting, by definition, means the guideline of nourishment consumption by not ingesting anything between real meals. Additionally, by the word intermittent, it pursues that a successive request of eating design must be achieved.

There's an assumption among specialists that the premise on how intermittent fasting functions can be clarified because of life systems and physiology; or the investigation of the organ and organ frameworks in connection to their capacities inside our bodies. As defined by experts, for example, doctors, inside our cerebrum stem lies the seat of satiety, yearning, and thirst called the nerve center. The nerve center is a complex, heterogeneous organ which arranges our body when to want to eat.

Subsequently, ought to there be any craving for man to drink or eat; the nerve center is the one in charge of such activity. Hence, whenever left untrained and left to do without anyone else will, satiety and appetite will increment to large extents.

When this occurs, the inclination to drink or eat will likewise be amplified. There is no peril or hazard to eating. There is nothing amiss with that; notwithstanding, the nature of the sustenance consumption we eat additionally decides the condition of wellbeing among people. Moreover, if a person continually ingests foods that are not nutritious, say the one we find in fast foods or cafeterias; and done in huge sums, wellbeing is influenced. Uncontrolled eating can prompt a large group of sicknesses, for example, diabetes, hypertension, cardiac or heart issues, and weight.

The ideal approach to begin your fasting is to design your meals deliberately. Intermittent fasting works best if it is done routinely and continuously. This fasting diet to get thinner must be done as per the eagerness of the member and must be trained to accomplish the ideal impacts. Besides fasting, if you intend to get thinner, the measure of caloric admission should likewise be considered. Along these lines, besides cautiously arranging the intermittent meals, the action of calories should also be mulled over.

Joining the two techniques won't merely make you thin; it will enable you to get the weight you've always needed. Additionally, preparing your nerve center to eat intermittently will hugely affect your desire to eat or drink which would prompt controlling your unfortunate dietary patterns.

Intermittent Fasting Can Be Beneficial For Your Body

Regardless of whether you will likely lose some genuinely significant weight or to get out your framework, intermittent fasting has many advantages for the body. The main thing I have to clear up is that fasting isn't equivalent to starving. Indeed, while the facts demonstrate that fasting implies not eating, intermittent fasting is completed a little at any given moment.

About Fasting

Fasting is a flawlessly standard part of life and has been accomplished for many years, for some reason. Fasting is utilized today in many active eating routine projects. People become overweight when they devour a more significant number of calories than they consume in a similar measure of time. With the inactive ways of life many of us lead, this has become typical. Fortunately, many incredible rec centers, weight reduction, and exercise programs exist to help with the issue of being overweight. Tragically, many can't bear the cost of or discover an opportunity to fit these into their bustling ways of life. Intermittent fasting can be beneficial for these people needing to get thinner.

The Benefits of Fasting

Despite what we do it a life all the time, it's in every case great to "take a vacation day" from it. The equivalent can be said for eating. A ton of garbage and destructive poisons go into our bodies every day. By taking a vacation day (intermittent fasting), we're allowing our bodies to dispose of these unsafe and extravagant things. Drinking a lot of water while you're fasting will help make it simpler and will wash down the body.

People that intermittent training fasting has discovered that they feel more beneficial and have a general better wellbeing. Intermittent fasting has many advantages for the body; the first is discharging out the shape for one day without anything returning into it. Besides, your body will encounter improved insulin resistance, which has a significant impact in many functions including better execution, muscle gain, weight reduction, sickness aversion, hostile to maturing and only a superior invulnerable framework as a rule.

When fasting is terrifying to you, you'll rapidly alter your perspective when you see the many advantages it accommodates your body and in general wellbeing. There is nobody approach to do intermittent fasting. Similarly, as with anything new, you need to do what works best for your way of life and individual propensities. Make irregular fasting a piece of your life, and you'll before long observe the advantages, with the first being you'll feel good. While you're fasting for one day, you'll be detoxifying and purifying out your body, without supplanting the things you're attempting to dispose of. It's a success win circumstance for your organization.

Intermittent Fasting - 5 Advantages of

Intermittent Fasting

Intermittent fasting is winding up increasingly more mainstream as a weight reduction and wellbeing the board device. It has a few significant points of interest over different methodologies. Here are five of them.

1: Counting calories is superfluous on intermittent fasting. Practically all dietary methodologies include tallying calories. While this might be essential after these transient eating plans, it is almost painful to do this long haul. This implies when the "diet" is finished, the classical rebound fat gain is practically around the bend after a time of unbendingly controlling all food.

2: You don't need to go hungry on intermittent fasting. When you are eating all your daily calories in a window of a few hours, it turns out to be substantially more hard to gorge when contrasted with a customary touching methodology. If you are fasting, you are not agonizing over whether a bite is alright or not. Fasting isn't eating, and when you break the quick, you eat if you are eager. Straightforward!

3: Your body doesn't attempt to hold tight to its fat stores when intermittent fasting. Most dietary methodologies are mostly prohibitive. Your body is for all time denied enough food and response be going into starvation mode. It holds tight to all your fat stores and hinders your digestion, precisely the opposite we need. When you can eat to satisfaction similar to the case on a fasting diet, your body responds by proceeding to drop body fat.

4: An intermittent fasting diet is less prohibitive than different weight control plans. Give us a chance to come to the heart of the matter here, and if your concept of good food is a burger and fries, nothing is going to help you until you change your discernment. It is consummately conceivable and even supportive of having some slack in what you eat. Without a doubt, begin with your protein and veggies. However, some of what you like makes them intrigue and positive hormonal impacts if you are endeavoring to get slender or even form some muscle.

5: An intermittent fasting diet adjusts to you. This is the pure magnificence of this methodology. Rather than attempting to discover precisely the correct number of grams of carbs or whatever at 10 am, you accommodated you are daily quick to your life and objectives. Some see a 16 hour fast from night until the following day at noon works best. Others favor a 24-hour cycle or even a 4-hour eating window. These are conceivable and have various focal points. It is a way of life as opposed to an eating regimen.

Best Weight Loss Drinks for Good And Healthy Diet

Did you realize that there are weight loss drinks that are as compelling in weight loss as other further developed methodologies? The discourse about getting in shape is ruled by which sustenance to maintain a strategic distance from or the amount to eat. The more significant part of the foods recommended achieving the undertaking by consuming the calories in the body through expanded digestion. The drinks proposed here pursue a similar weight loss system of improving digestion, an activity that is in profound stand out from the event of the regular sugary and carbonated refreshments.

As indicated by an exploration done by the American diary of clinical nourishment, higher milk admission can altogether help in your diet. Working with an example populace of grown-ups for a time of as long as two years, the specialists found checked weight loss in milk takers, with some losing as much as 12 pounds toward the finish of the trial. The refreshment is a rich wellspring of calcium which is utilized for the breakdown of fat cells. The nearness of no small measure of protein in milk may likewise help in lessening irregular eating along these lines overseeing cases of weight gain. Include some little rules of the beverage in your dinners for expanded consuming of muscle to fat ratio.

Yogurt is a milk item and very compelling for weight reduction as well. Nutritionists believe the beverage to be super sustenance on account of its wealth in minerals and nutrients that guide in many body capacities, including digestion. Passing by an investigation directed by the international journey of heftiness in 2005, there is an explanation behind overweight individuals to consider yogurt in their dietary weight loss programs. Utilizing fat-free yogurt on fat grown-ups, it was found that the individuals who included fat-free yogurt recorded more weight loss than the individuals who depended on other calorie-cutting strategies as it were. Counting a few servings of yogurt in your daily diet may, therefore, enhance weight loss due to less craving, and expanded calcium in the body.

Even though the connection between expanded water admission and dieting is still under research, the discoveries there is proof that taking an adequate measure of the beverage prompts diminished sustenance craving, want for vegetables and natural products, and expanded copying of calories in the body. As much as drinking water supposedly is powerful in weight the board, dietitians always exhortation patients not to substitute their diet with water as this may prompt broad wellbeing outcomes. To decrease the hunger for sustenance and control calories consumption, it is prudent to drink some water before each dinner. This technique has additionally been viewed as a successful method for upgrading the consuming of calories and would, therefore, be useful for your diet.

Green tea admission is generally connected with the board of cancerous growth and other related conditions. Its superb enemy of oxidant properties could likewise be used in weight the executives particularly for the end of fats. Consider drinking around four glasses of the refreshments for fast reduction of the muscle versus fat.

Likewise to be considered for weight loss is an organic grape product whose causticity is thought to add to extraordinary weight reduction impacts. The juice works best when it is customarily extricated. The weight loss drinks referenced here are regular at home and could shape viable solutions for weight the board.

CHAPTER NINE

INTERMITTENT FASTING FOR SUGGESTIONS

Intermittent fasting includes rotating you're eating design between times of fasting (expending just water) and non-fasting (eating). The eating times can be a real factor and stretch out more than a few days. A portion of the more drawn out non-eating periods incorporates a 36-hour quick pursued by 12 hours of eating (generally broken into three meals around 3-4 hours separated) Most intermittent fasting diets stretch out over 24 hours, enabling the individual to remain predictable from every day. The more forceful of these day-long fasts limit an individual to 4 hours of eating (as a rule during the evening). The most broadly acknowledged fasting routine includes an 8-hour window for eating.

Intermittent fasting has been considered broadly on the two creatures and people. Except if the quick was reached out past 36 hours, no negative impacts were seen in the guineas pigs (other than gentle to direct appetite torments). Intermittent fasting has been appeared to decrease body fat, stabilize blood sugars, and increment muscle reaction.

How can it work? Everything rotates around the hormone insulin. Your body discharges insulin at whatever point you expend sustenance (all the more so for nourishments high in starches). The insulin invigorates the retention of nutrients (for the most part glucose) into your fat and muscle tissue. Since more often than not the muscle cells are not vitality denied, overabundance nutrients after meals are put away in your fat mass (glucose is likewise put away as glycogen in your liver). It takes around 3 hours after supper times before your body's insulin level drops to pre-dinner levels. At the lower insulin fixations, your liver and fat tissue discharge the put away glucose and fatty acids into your bloodstream for vitality. By broadening the time between meals, you increment the length of this catabolic state when your body consumes off fat.

If you were advised to eat 5-6 small meals every day? Visit dinner utilization impedes the body's fat-consuming procedure. Under a comparable diet, an individual utilizing an intermittent fasting approach will accomplish a lower body fat rate than the constant eater. Remember, that the nature of your diet is progressively significant that the planning. Intermittent fasting isn't a reason for gorging on low-quality nourishment later around evening time.

Despite everything, you have to eat clean. Besides, you will need to build your protein utilization when on a fasting diet. Protein is the best macronutrient as far as satiety, implying that calorie-for-calorie, the protein will stifle the sentiment of yearning for longer than will sugars or fats. Eating a high-protein/low-carb diet is an absolute necessity, particularly on non-exercise days.

Discontinuous Fasting to Get Rid of Back Fat - What is Fasting and How Do You Benefit from It?

Wellness fans frequently are discussing 'intermittent fasting' while talking about weight reduction and fat misfortune techniques. What is intermittent fasting and what you ought to do to dispose of back fat utilizing fasting technique?

Intermittent fasting is a compelling apparatus for perpetual fat misfortune. However, it is critical to remember that everyone ought to alter his fasting convention to accommodate his body parameters to dispose of his back fat as fast as would be prudent. Consequences of fasting are impacted by individual's volume of preparing and other physical exercises, recuperation capacity and examples, diet macronutrient proportions, practice program type, dietary patterns and way of life, current body creation and everyday way of life. That implies you should begin with essential fasting project and screen your outcomes. At that point, you can change the program to accommodate your body needs to boost disposing of back fat.

The aftereffects of intermittent fasting are not constrained to fat misfortune. Intermittent fasting can result in an increase of slender bulk, wellbeing and execution upgrades, better processing of sustenance, improved insusceptible capacity additionally. A significant benefit of fasting is improved insulin obstruction which is the establishment of fat misfortune impact of fasting and digestion improvement.

Fasting by definition is the demonstration of going without sustenance and drinks or nourishment for a certain period, ordinarily somewhere in the range of 8 and 72 hours. Intermittent fasting is joining 16-24 hour long fasts of into your way of life. It very well may be done day by day or a few times each week relying upon the length of fast. Amid intermittent fast you are not expending any sustenance, however, you are as yet drinking sans calorie drinks like water, espresso, or tea without sugar, flavor, and whatever other added substances which may contain calories.

It is encouraged to begin fasting gradually. At first, you should start with 1-2 times each week with fasts of 18-20 hours. For instance, you can have your supper today at 8 PM and afterward fast till 2 PM tomorrow around lunchtime. Drink heaps of water amid the fast. You can include a touch of lemon juice or apple juice vinegar to your water. Espresso and tea are likewise OK as referenced previously. At that point, at 2 PM you can break your fast with a typical supper you would have during this time just if you would not have fasted. Congrats! You have finished your first intermittent fast!

Intermittent fasting is a basic, yet viable technique for losing fat and particularly for disposing of your back fat. The main concern you have to do is to decay any sustenance for a predetermined period. We suggest starting with one quick for 18 hours out of consistently and after that including second quick of

18 hours in 2-3 weeks.

Will Intermittent Fasting Help You Lose Weight

In specific situations, there is a lot of proof that says intermittent fasting can help with consuming fat. Intermittent fasting is dividing your last dinner of the day and your first feast the following day more remote separated to as much as 16 hours. The objective is that after you eat, your body takes around six to eight hours to utilize that glycogen, at that point to keep working it goes into your fat stores.

If we begin bolstering our body before that six to eight timeframe, or before the glycogen has been utilized, we never enable our framework to take advantage of our fat stockpiling. This makes it hard to ever get in shape. We can go too far when we quick. When we go past a specific point, our framework acknowledges it won't get any more nourishment and goes into starvation mode. By then it fundamentally quits utilizing our abundance fat.

Tests have appeared there are extra medical advantages to intermittent fasting. These incorporate expanding insulin sensitivity, lessening oxidative stress, and increment the limit with regards to opposing cell stress. These will hinder maturing of the phones just as avoiding ailments related to cell harm.

So is an intermittent fasting plan directly for everybody? The majority of the variables that go into healthy weight decrease make it about trying to discover one enchantment slug that will be straight for everybody. To start with, it is protected to state that pregnant ladies should never quick. An infant needs every one of the supplements they can get, and a few examinations have proposed that fasting can adjust the infant's pulse and breathing examples, alongside expanding gestational diabetes.

Those that experience the ill effects of hypoglycemia, a state of the unusually lower dimension of glucose, ought not to experience times of fasting. Your objective if you have this condition is standardized your glucose levels first, at that point if you choose to settle on a less unbending variant of fasting quickly. Those with diabetes likewise won't be assisted with intermittent fasting.

At long last, you should understand that when you are going excessively quick, you should give considerably more consideration to your nutrition levels when you do eat. By proceeding with a poisonous rich diet of exceptionally handled nourishments, at that point continue to not eat for 15 or 16 hours, you could be making your body more mischief than anything over the long haul. Assembling a healthy diet plan to ensure you are getting the proper nutrition in the shorter timespan you are eating it will be fundamental.

At whatever point you are going to roll out dramatic improvements in your diet, regardless of whether they are healthy changes that will in the long run extraordinarily advantage your wellbeing, it might take a short time for your framework to conform to the change. However, tune in to what your body is letting you know, and if you are going excessively rapidly, don't battle it. Go a bit slower with the changes, and if it is useful for your framework will in the long run adjust.

Standard Fasting Could Help You Live Longer

Standard fasting could turn into the most recent wellbeing furor after research uncovered it's useful to get in shape, yet could be helpful for the body and increment future!

Relevant research has demonstrated that standard fasting can enable you to shed pounds, consume painful muscle to fat ratio, and usually support development hormone. In any case, by investigating down this new heading of life span makes it significantly all the more engaging for health food nuts, as regular fasting could likewise enable them to live more.

Generally, keeping the body from sustenance has been viewed as a type of discipline, bound to be related to religious practices or, in its extraordinary structure, with a dietary issue, for example, anorexia.

A developing collection of proof proposes that avoiding nourishment for 24 hours on regular events, be it week after week or month to month, can convey a large group of remedial characteristics.

For instance, it was discovered that asthma patients who fasted routinely, had a couple of manifestations and demonstrated preferred aviation route work over those that did not.

Then again, the goliath nourishment and diet industry continue endeavoring to persuade everybody that to get in shape you should continue eating! As indicated by them, transient fasting does not diminish fat consuming catalysts. Furthermore, the risk of brief times of intermittent fasting could go into starvation mode, and quit getting more fit?

It could be contended notwithstanding, that their recommendation could be inclination and affected by the loss of income. Relevant research demonstrates that the exact inverse occurs. Transient fasting does in truth 'expands' the action of fat consuming proteins.

Nutrition specialists leading exploration on the metabolic impacts of brief times of fasting in people and its potential application in weight reduction could direct various body organization tests on numerous competitors and top dimension muscle heads. Observing them while they ate less and attempted new exploratory health improvement plans

A large number of the analyses led had results that were altogether different based on what was reasonable, and the acknowledgment that to comprehend the nutrition job in weight reduction, they would need to begin from the earliest starting point and study the result for the body when it abandons any nourishment.

In an exploration consider distributed in the diary of Sports Science and Medicine, ten world-class control competitors were inspected previously, amid and following 30 days of intermittent fasting.

The scientists found that there was no drop in execution amid their fasts or even in the days after their 30-day fasting period. Genuinely fantastic considering they were all top competitors.

The advantages of regular fasting for good wellbeing and weight reduction has created very differing suppositions dependent on the most recent outcomes, and similarly, as with much dietary exhortation, conclusions are isolated. While a few specialists think fasting is a more straightforward method to control calorie consumption than delayed confinements on exceptional eating regimens, others caution against it.

Fasting may not be for everybody. The science behind viably starving yourself is associated with how the body uses glucose; however, precisely why it gave such medical advantages is as yet open for the hypothesis.

Data contained in this part isn't intended to supplant expert guidance. Continuously check with your doctor before beginning any weight reduction or fasting program.

CHAPTER TEN

INTERMITTENT FASTING FOR FAT LOSS: GOOD OR BAD?

As you might have noticed, my title for this article includes a quite sweet wit if I should state. Today I needed to remember the present time of year, Holidays. With that in mind, lets first take a quick minute to be thankful for all or a portion of the following. Your vehicle, your cash, your personality, your image among friends and associates, your shoes, your new cool tech gadget and all other cool things we consume. Or then again I surmise we can say goodness yea, cool it on all that and be thankful for friends, family, friends and family, wellbeing, rooftops over our head, incredible opportunities, extraordinary and inexhaustible food, clean water, and a fantastic general community.

When we remember a portion of the above, it puts into perspective the stuff that we spread here every week. Presently I would prefer not to diminish the importance of this information by any stretch of the imagination, yet more so placed it in its proper spot to make beyond any doubt that we as a whole realize it is not an incomprehensibly important issue but instead that it is something that can be utilized to increase your general quality of life in such vast numbers of ways. Furthermore, subsequently helping you bring more to the community you are a piece of.

Intermittent FASTING 101:

You could conceivably have known about Intermittent Fasting. It is a somewhat simple nutritional intervention that is being widely utilized and rather effectively might I include. It involves splitting your 24 hour day into two necessary states or categories.

"Fast"- ed or "Fast"- ing state: (Anywhere from 18-48 hours)

"Sustained" or "Feed"- ing state

Let us take a gander at your fasting state first. The time ranges from 16 to 48 hours. I have played with the 16-hour state as of late and have had a couple of experiences with the 24 hours fast too.

To begin this off, you will typically have your dinner around lets state 7 or 8 pm. You would then enter your Fast for the next 16-18 hours for this example. So, you would then get up the following day and potentially have your morning workout or prepare for work.

Side note: If you work out in the mornings, I would not do this on workout days but instead 1 x for every week. I lean toward this on days of cardio just or 1 x for every week of Resistance Training workouts.

You would then take a gander at consuming your first meal around 11 am - 1 pm of that day.

Things to consider during your fast:

Potential Irritability

Increased need for water consumption

More prominent ability to differentiate between false hunger and genuine hunger

Incredible caloric deficit and resetting of the body's fat burning hormonal environment.

Need for the consumption of Amino Acids during "fasting state" (specifically when morning "fasted state" workouts.)

Increased need for a delicious adjusted meal when you happen to the fasted state.

Presently let us take a gander at the Feed-ing state.

This time will last the next 6-10 hours, depending on your last meal during the current day. During this time it is advisable to consume your main 3 meals. You still eat aka (Break the Fast) exactly sometime in the not too distant future than your ordinary routine. It doesn't need to include your typical breakfast food yet definitely can if that your thing.

Every meal will be of a decent size and will prop you up securely into the next day.

Things to consider during your Feed-ing or Fed state:

If you workout in the evening has a go at keeping carbs moderate to low for pre-workout meals and afterward have a substantial carb meal after your evening workout to finish off the day and resulting in the sustained state.

Don't go insane on shoddy nourishment for your first meal after the fast that will thoroughly eradicate all great coming from the fast.

Have the meals be of customary size and portions. Listen to your body and dependably take into consideration 15-20 minutes after eating to check whether you need more food. That is to what extent it typically takes a meal to achieve your belly and its tangible receptors that signal hunger.

Pros and Cons of Intermittent Fasting + General Guidelines:

Pro: Create a massive caloric deficit

Pro: Increases fat and calorie burning

Pro: Increases ability to recognize genuine and bogus faculties of hunger

Pro: You don't need to eat each 2-3 hours which can be a pain in the bum

Pro: Increased vitality levels and metabolism

Cons: Women experience severe difficulties with this diet

Cons: Takes a little getting used to

Cons: You may feel level at times however that is not frequently detailed

Guidelines:

I don't recommend this more than 2-4 x weekly with 2-3 days being the sweet spot for me now.

I recommend you give it a shot and perceive how you react to it. Each body is different.

Have some amino acids close by and be ready to take those during your morning hours and previously/after workouts.

Ultimately dependably consult with your medical specialist before attempting this.

There you have it, folks. Give this intermittent fasting for fat misfortune an attempt and offer your musings and comments with me as it generally encourages me to make this stuff progressively simplified for you when I get those comments and questions.

Intermittent Fasting Vs Low Carb Diet?

If you are searching for a way to reduce your body fat, going low carb is one of the prevalent diet decisions — there various adaptations of low carb diets, from the renowned Atkins diet toward The South Beach Diet. Low Carb Diets are not new. Dr. Robert Atkins did not develop the idea, the same number of individuals assume. Low Carb diets even go before different U.S. diet specialists, for example, Herman Tarnower and Herman Taller. Dieting Plans allowing you to eat meat, some dairy foods, a plate of mixed greens and non-starchy vegetables, while limiting or forbidding foods containing sugar or starch were first advanced in the mid-nineteenth century by Jean Anthelme Brillat-Savarin. Right up 'til the present time the discussion proceeds among Doctors and Nutritionists concerning what is the best diet for us to follow and lose weight.

There is positive proof to demonstrate that underlying weight loss while following a low carb diet reduces body fat. In an ongoing study of popular diets (Gardner CD, Kiazand An, Alhassan S, et al. Examination of the Atkins, Zone, Ornish, and LEARN diets for change in weight and related hazard factors among overweight premenopausal ladies: the A TO Z Weight Loss Study: a randomized preliminary. JAMA 2007;297:969-77) The Atkins diet demonstrated the best weight loss results over both a 2 month and 6 months. This is the data you see referenced in the media all the time. Anyway, over 12 months, the Atkins diet results were not all that amazing and were not any more effective than different diets in the study.

My view dependent on my experience of attempting low carb dieting is however useful for the time being, diets, for example, Atkins is not reasonable to follow in the long term. As I would like to think, to lose body fat and control weight, the way we eat must be conceivable to follow as long as possible, not only for a couple of weeks. I have in the past done Atkins, The South Beach Diet, and Fat Flush. I have taken things from these diet plans. I use them as a significant aspect of lifestyle today. I additionally have a greater comprehension of the impact refined carbohydrates have on my body. However, the straightforward certainty remains I couldn't follow these plans as a long-term lifestyle change.

This year I turned into a Retired Dieter. This implies I never again will won't eat the foods I enjoy. I have quit tuning in to the media talk about the most recent new diet and fat loss furor. All diets have a snare, however toward the day's end it boils down to a specific something, somehow, we need to eat less. So, what is the arrangement?

For me, the effective way to lose body fat, and control my weight, is by utilizing intermittent Fasting. Intermittent Fasting is just taking occasions of fast (no food) and working them into your lifestyle. Despite everything you eat each day, however, you will incorporate a period of up to 24hrs without food into your day. Utilizing Intermittent Fasting a few times per week reduces body fat, yet still allows you to enjoy the foods you enjoy. On the days you are not fasting, you eat typically. Following the I.F.

lifestyle, I am as yet cutting carbs from my diet. I am cutting carbs for what might be compared to 2 entire days out of every week.

We could discuss the hypothesis, yet I like to take a shot at results. In my initial 7 weeks of utilizing Intermittent Fasting for weight loss, I have reduced my body fat by 12% and lost 24lbs. In my 14 years of attempting different diet plans, I have never had results that contrast with these. The other central matter is, not ordinary for my experience of low carb diets.

I have not felt confined with Intermittent Fasting; I have not had any yearnings for specific foods as I did with Low Carb dieting because no foods are untouchable. For what reason do I feel that intermittent Fasting is something I can use them as long term after just 7 weeks?

The appropriate response is because on any diet I have attempted in the past, I would always have days where I believed I was limited, so the diet ended up trying, and that is on the diets that I figured out how to stick to for 7 weeks! The difference with Intermittent Fasting is, is anything but a diet because no foods are beyond reach.

When you have finished once fast, you know from that day forward, you can incorporate it into your lifestyle, how you do that, and how frequently you do it, is up to you, that is the excellent thing about Intermittent Fasting, it adjusts to your lifestyle, in the past when you stopped eating so much junk food, how regularly did it command your life? This again is a prime model why diets fizzle.

So, my recommendation is if you are hoping to reduce your body fat, and figure you ought to cut your carbs, attempt Intermittent Fasting. Become a Retired Dieter, and let me know how you jump on.

How Can I Lose A Stone In A Month - Rapid Weight Loss With Intermittent Fasting

Fast Yet Sustained Weight Loss

1 month, 1 stone, 1 coordinated exertion

Let's figure out what's essential to accomplish this. If we accept 30 days for a month, at that point we need to lose about 5lbs every 10 days (about 2kg, or 15lb in 3o days, or 0.5lb/day, or over 3lbs every week).

I'm going to take an imaginary man and woman and put a few figures down for them, showing you how to do it for yourself if you're different from my models.

If we expect that there are around 3500 calories in a pound of fat, at that point, you need to create a shortfall of in any event 11500 calories every week, if you need to get those 3lbs off (3500 x 14lbs = 49000cals).

If we at that point separate that into every day, that is a day by day shortfall of around 1600 calories.

Presently, how about we find out how much energy it expenses to remain to live:

I'll take 3 men and 3 ladies.

Male 1

70kg - 11st 0.3lb - 154.3lbs

Energy cals (range) 1,918 - 3,036

Male 2

80kg - 12st 8.4lb - 176.4lbs

Energy cals (range) 2,038 - 3,226

Male 3

90kg - 14st 2.4lb - 198.4lbs

Energy cals (range) 2,158 - 3,416

Female 1

60kg - 9st 6.3lb - 132.3lbs

Energy cals (range) 1,598 - 2,531

Female 2

70kg - 11st 0.3lb - 154.3lbs

Energy cals (range) - 1,718 - 2,721

Female 3

80kg - 12st 8.4lb - 176.4lbs

Energy cals (range) - 1,838 - 2,911

Notes: The ranges appeared day by day calorie expenditure are dependent on movement level, from sedentary (think office worker that drives to work and takes no or extremely restricted exercise) to highly dynamic (somebody who has an activity that includes a few hours of exhausting work every day, or exercises for in excess of 90 mins at a high intensity/reliably high pulse every day).

These imaginary figures depend on somebody being about 170cm tall, in their mid 30's, and are used for delineation purposes, the standards behind the practices here are substantial, you need to personalize the exercises to your circumstance. These are estimations and will differ person to person, to find out more precisely you need to get your starting figures. You can do this using the calculators found at caloriesperhour.com. Use the BMR and RMR calcs for a rough starting point; at that point, use the practices here to modify the figures dependent on certifiable results.

So you can see that for a woman of 60kg, who is just lightly dynamic or stationary, this would mean not eating by any stretch of the imagination, for about a month!

Who is this for? Thing is though, and a 60kg woman doesn't generally need to lose 14lbs (about 6kg) or over 10% of her body weight, so we're not by any stretch of the imagination catering for this person. What we ought to take a gander at is the higher end of the scale. That is the place big weight loss numbers are convenient.

If, for instance, you take a gander at the 90kg man, even a sedentary individual could cut more than 1000 cals from their day by day consumption, as long as they do it with the right foods. I'll hit on that in a minute.

Initially, how about we investigate the 3 factors that will make this large calorie decrease conceivable.

Intermittent Fasting

Eating high protein, low fat, low carb.

Doing just high-intensity weights and exceptionally low-intensity cardio.

Presently how about we grow each of those so you can create your very own plan.

1: Intermittent Fasting

Intermittent Fasting (the Leangains rendition) is a simple

approach to feeding the body. You split the day into two phases, an eating phase, and a non-eating phase. The eating phase keeps going around 8 hours; in this manner, the fasting phase endures about 16 hours. This doesn't imply that you eat for the entire of the 8-hour block!

There are two key viewpoints to IF that make it work to support you with regards to enormous weight loss.

1: Each day is split, physiologically, into two distinct phases, every one of which helps your fat loss goal. These two phases are an anabolic, or tissue building phase, and fat burning, or energy breakdown phase.

2: Using IF makes it a lot simpler to diminish your calories than conventional dieting.

I don't need to go into more insight regarding the IF lifestyle, because you can peruse the two posts on my website (address at base, scan the Intermittent Fasting Category for 'Intermittent Fasting Results and Guide' and 'Training For Fat Loss') that recount to the full story, do the trick to state, if you need to make your weight loss as easy and powerful as could be expected under the circumstances, you ought to presumably be doing some IF.

2: Eating High Protein, Low Fat, Low Carb

In his brilliant arrangement of articles about designing a fat loss diet, Lyle MacDonald discusses setting things up from the ground, as opposed to the top. State what? All things considered, what we've done here is started with a weight loss goal, that being the top or end point, and the worked in reverse to figure out what we need to do. Lyle adopts a slightly different strategy and figures out what you need physiologically, and after that puts those figures into a diet, to perceive what turns out toward the end. Here, we are going to use some portion of that approach (setting protein admission) to give you a starting point for figuring out your foods.

What amount of food do you need?

Or on the other hand more specifically, what amount of protein would it be advisable for you to go for at every meal? Indeed, we can give two answers to that question, and the best solution is the one that makes you feel generally consoled. The quick answer is 'lots.' The more specific answer is worked out as follows; start with a level of about 1g/lb of bodyweight and gap over your a few meals, and after that modify dependent on fit tissue and strength drops and hunger/satiety levels. So if you find your strength dropping, and your muscle leaving your body, you need to add more protein in, and if you find yourself getting hungry between meals or not satisfied at a meal, add more protein!

What Foods Can I Eat?

I've assembled a rundown of foods that will work while eating for substantial fat loss. You can download it from my website, using the connection at the base. One thing that I reliably find is the total lack of hunger and feelings of hardship when on this kind of diet, and this shouldn't astonish given the massive range of foods on offer here. One thing you'll notice is the total lack of liquid foods/meal replacement powders/protein drinks. This is purposeful; they don't give satiety and fulfillment, and they don't offer much open door for long term diet adherence. As Martin Berkhan says, 'don't drink your calories.'

Why High Protein, Low Fat, Low Carb?

Two or three reasons; 1, you need to keep calories as low as could be allowed, as quickly as would be prudent. 2, protein, in addition to lots of massive yet small carb thickness foods, gives the most straightforward way to feel full, satisfied, and cheerful when cutting calories.

3: Doing just high-intensity weights and exceptionally low-intensity cardio

Every one of the three segments in this weight loss plan is similarly significant, so you would be wise to find a way of including this part! Inquire as to whether it merits jeopardizing the entire procedure for missing some simple exercises?

Why start with an announcement like that?

Because it's unreasonably simple for some people to drop once more into old ways of 'exercising for weight loss.'

What you NEED to do is overwhelming weights, with low reps and using as significant developments as could reasonably be expected. Keep in mind, big weights are precise to every person, and the exact number/weight is excessive, what's significant is that you lift to YOUR ability and you figure out how to completely lift at your ability. For those of you that have barely lifted weights before that implies learning what a maximum exertion lift feels like, AND expecting that maximum to go up rapidly as you figure out how to get increasingly more out of yourself.

The great thing about this program is that it truly is simple. Take the following exercises and turn them:

Squat

Dumbell press, seat press or bodyweight dips

Dumbell or free weight shoulder press

Lat pulldown, pullup, seated column or twisted around free weight/dumbell push

Deadlift.

Your pivot is simple: Do 3 weeks of 5set of 4-6 reps (5x5 style schedule) and after that 3 weeks of 3 sets of 9-12 reps (3x10 style schedule). Each time you hit the higher rep range, you increment the weight. Simply following 10-14 weeks do you need to rest (however if you've just been exercising reliably for over 12 weeks, you need to take a week of total rest right now - except if your goal is inside 12 weeks from the start of your program, in which case, you get your rest toward the end of that!)

If you don't have a clue how to do these exercises, you can get guidance from a capable mentor (you can find if they're any good by watching how they get you to move and concentrate on the exercises your learning, if they get you to do your exercises like those done in guidance recordings you might make sure they know their stuff), or you can look at the bountiful measure of vids on YouTube and figure your specific manner.

George 'Super BootCamps' Harris is a Personal Trainer, Hypnotherapist, Master NLP Practitioner, Certified Strength, and Conditioning Specialist, and Nutritional Coach.

George composed his ebook, 'How To Do What You Don't Want To Do' to help people assume responsibility for their capacity to persuade themselves, feel good and get results from their diet and exercise. Composed for everybody to quickly comprehend and apply, this book contains everything you need to assume responsibility for your motivation and get results.

With this book you can at long last end the cycle of motivation and hopelessness, be predictable and learn - quickly - how to feel good about doing exercise, how to make dieting simple and make yourself feel good whenever.

CONCLUSION

Getting in shape isn't that troublesome. It is straightforward. For a great many people this may sound outlandish, and they may believe this is a falsehood. However, it's most certainly not. Shedding a couple of pounds and picking up muscle in the meantime in half a month isn't a fantasy. How? It's not the drunk over the top eating regimens. It's not the costly uncommon and nutritious enhancements or nourishment. It's not the eat-little dinners six-times-every day program. It's no of those programs which don't guarantee a ton for a real existence time program. Try not to be amazed, yet the appropriate response is in intermittent fasting.

This may sound ludicrous to specific individuals, however for inquiries about this isn't a joke. Explores on transient fasting or intermittent fasting have indicated what an incredible program it is, and to be placed at the top of the priority list, it isn't the equivalent with eating routine prevailing fashions. By doing flexible intermittent fasting, there is no requirement for starvation or slobbering like distraught at a glimpse of tasty sustenance. It is adaptable, so it won't prevent you from eating your preferred food. The examination led demonstrated this purported fasting will build the harmful chemical in the body in this way individuals will get more fit much more straightforward by not working more enthusiastically. That is the general purpose of doing this program. It's the least demanding and quickest method for getting in shape. Quit buckling down with weight loss programs that are not giving you the outcome you should get. With intermittent fasting, don't stress over vitality. Many individuals who have been doing transient fasting demonstrate that they feel empowered and most profitable when they are fasting. This is because fasting does not influence your digestion.